MENINGITIS

A GUIDE FOR FAMILIES

Meningitis- a guide for families
is published by Publishing Solutions (U.K.) Ltd.
Unit 6A Alston Works, Alston Road, Barnet,
Herts. EN5 4EL.

Cover illustration
The cover illustration is based on a
photomicrograph of meningococcal bacteria and
was kindly provided by M H Thompson

About the authors
The authors are paediatricians at Imperial
College School of Medicine at St Mary's
Hospital in London. Simon Kroll is the
Professor of Paediatrics and Molecular
Infectious Diseases, Andrew Pollard is the
Action Research Fellow, and Parviz Habibi is
Senior Lecturer and Director of the Paediatric
Intensive Care Unit. All three are parents
themselves.

Printed in Great Britain by
Redwood Books, Trowbridge, Wiltshire.

ISBN No.: 1-901336-00-X

MENINGITIS
A GUIDE FOR FAMILIES

by

J Simon Kroll MA MRCPCH FRCP
Andrew J Pollard BSc MRCPCH MRCP
Parviz Habibi PhD MRCPCH FRCP

Department of Paediatrics
Imperial College School of Medicine at St Mary's Hospital
London W2 1PG

To families everywhere

Contents

Foreword

I recommend this book to all parents.

There are some 2,000 cases of meningococcal disease each year in the UK, and whether you regard this as a rare or a common disease, it is one of which we are all rightfully fearful.

These pages provide an easily accessible account of meningitis in general and meningococcal disease in particular. They contain twelve real life stories with vivid colour photographs which portray meningococcal disease in all its forms, from a flu-like illness to a fulminating spotted fever. While medical cases like these are of interest to some, they are of importance to all of us. Understanding a health problem goes some way towards alleviating our fears. However in the case of meningococcal disease, armed with knowledge about its presentation can lead to early action which can make the difference between life and death.

From this book you will learn when to call for emergency medical help: you will understand the value of early antibiotic treatment: and you will see how critical admission to a fully equipped Paediatric Intensive Care Unit can be.

It is appropriate that this book has been written this year, which marks the 200th anniversary of Edward Jenner's first vaccination against smallpox. As you will read, vaccination trials against meningococcal disease are even now at the experimental stage and justify hope for the extinction of meningococcal disease in the near future.

Meanwhile we must protect our children today by early recognition of the symptoms and signs of meningococcal disease and by decisive action.

On behalf of all parents I should like to express my indebtedness to the St Mary's team for writing this book and for their pioneering work in the treatment of meningococcal disease and their research towards its final eradication.

Professor David Baum, President-elect,
Royal College of Paediatrics and Child Health.
Bristol, 10th December 1996.

Preface

The children's department at St Mary's Hospital in London specialises in the diagnosis and treatment of children's infections. Several times a week through the winter, patients are admitted to our children's wards and intensive care unit suffering from meningitis or septicaemia. Many make a complete recovery but sadly some die despite all that can be done. In every case families have been horrified by the speed with which their children have become desperately ill. They have been anxious to find out as much as they can about these conditions, and have wished that they had known something about them before hand.

Until now, there has been little suitable for family reading. While cases of meningitis attract a great deal of media attention, even though the disease is rare, much of what is published is in a sensational style that can be alarmist, inaccurate or both.

Our aim with this book is therefore simple. First and foremost, it is to provide the information that gives the best chance of recognising that a baby, child or adult might be developing the disease. In chapter 1, "Could it be meningitis?" we have described the way meningitis can develop, and also described the related and very serious condition of septicaemia. In chapter 2, "Case Histories", twelve true stories, told by victims or their parents, paint vivid pictures of the way in which these diseases can strike. In the rest of the book the conditions of meningitis and septicaemia are described in detail in answer to many questions we have been asked about these diseases, the germs that cause them, how they are spread, the way they are treated, the problems that can come in their wake, and how one day we may at last be able to prevent them.

In having written this book we may be criticised that we too are increasing anxiety about a rare condition, contributing to a state of panic, and needlessly increasing the work load of doctors in the community and in hospitals. However, all doctors agree that the early recognition of meningitis is vital, and this can only be achieved if the public has some understanding of the disease and the way it develops. We believe that parents should be well informed about all health matters so that they can take an active part in making health decisions for their children. We hope that with this book, we present the facts in a straight forward way that will inform rather than alarm.

We gratefully acknowledge the work of those parents and children who have been ready to share their stories, and dedicate this book to them, to all our meningitis families, and to the Meningitis Research Foundation in acknowledgement of the crucial part they play in the fight against meningitis and the support they give to families devastated by the disease.

Simon Kroll, Andrew J Pollard, Parviz Habibi.
London, 4th December 1996

Acknowledgments

We thank Professor David Baum for kindly agreeing to write the foreword, and our friends and colleagues - Alison and Sam Clarke (parents), Simon Currin (GP), Jane Garnett (parent), Pat Gubbins (director, Meningitis Research Foundation), Beverley Habibi (parent), Mark Herbert (paediatrician), Andrew and Carolyn Knight (GPs), Mary and William Kroll (mother and teenage son), Edward and Leah Ley-Wilson (parents), Neil MacLennan (GP) Teresa Munby (parent), Ralph and Lorna Ockendon (parents), Rachel Pollard (hospital doctor), Mary Ramsay (Public Health specialist), Ken Williamson (GP) - who kindly read parts or all of our book as it developed and suggested many improvements. Robert Gray's illustrations are gratefully acknowledged. We thank the Audio Visual Unit of Imperial College School of Medicine at St Mary's Hospital for permission to reproduce clinical photographs, and Mr M H Thompson of the Centre for Applied Microbiology and Research, Porton Down, for permission to use the photograph of meningococcal bacteria reproduced on the cover and on page 102. Figure 2 is reprinted from the Journal of Infection, vol 27(1): DM Jones and RH Mallard, "Age incidence of meningococcal infection, England and Wales 1984-1991" p 83-88 (1993), by permission of the publisher WB Saunders Co Ltd, London.

How to use this book

Whatever your interest in this book - whether you are concerned about meningitis from stories in the media, or whether you have personal or family experience of the disease - we recommend that you **read the Introduction, and then:**

- Concerned about recognising the disease in your child?
  Read chapters 1 and 2

- Interested in increasing your knowledge of meningitis:
  What is it? What causes it? Who gets it and why?
  How is it treated? What are the after-effects?
  Read chapters 3, 4, and 5 and the Conclusion

- Travelling and worried about the possibility of meningitis?
  Read Chapter 7

- Interested in prevention of meningitis, and vaccines?
  Read Chapters 6, 7 and 8

- Interested in the experiences of others, and in
  Support Groups
  Read Chapter 2 and the Appendix

- Baffled by a technical term?
  Check the Glossary

Introduction

Meningitis is a rare disease. Around 2000 cases are reported each year in England and Wales (population nearly 52 million), which means that a General Practioner (GP) might only see one or two cases in his/her entire career. Meningitis is a seasonal disease. Rather than being spread throughout the year, cases in the UK mainly occur in winter, and as Christmas approaches, meningitis stories hit the headlines. Meningitis is a terrifying disease. The speed with which people fall ill, and the dramatic and sometimes fatal course of infection, are so frightening that everyone wants to know what it is and how to recognise if a case is developing.

Some basic facts

Meningitis is a disease of the young in particular, more common in babies and toddlers than in older children and adults. It is an infection of the membranes surrounding the brain, which can be caused by different kinds of germs, including viruses and bacteria. The majority of cases are caused by viruses. Viral meningitis, though unpleasant, is not usually a severe illness. Meningitis caused by bacteria is less common, but much more serious. Three different kinds of bacteria are responsible for most cases of meningitis: meningococcal, pneumococcal and Hib bacteria. **The diagnosis of bacterial meningitis must be made quickly, and treatment in hospital must be given urgently.**

Children with bacterial meningitis may also have septicaemia (also known as blood poisoning), in which bacteria spread throughout the body in the bloodstream. Meningococcal bacteria, which are the commonest cause of bacterial meningitis, can cause very severe septicaemia. This can develop even without meningitis, and is much more dangerous. Meningitis and septicaemia are often confused in television and newspaper reports, especially when the cause is infection with meningococcal bacteria. Because in any case they may occur in the same patient at the same time, both diseases are considered in this book.

Excellent leaflets and posters are widely available for people to learn how to recognise meningitis. These stress the importance of well-known meningitis features - headache, dislike of bright lights, and stiff neck. Unfortunately, all of these signs and symptoms may be absent in someone with dangerous septicaemia. The signs and symptoms both of meningitis and of septicaemia are therefore described in detail in the next chapter of this book.

CHAPTER 1
Could it be meningitis?

Most parents have no difficulty recognising when their child is unwell, but when your child is ill with a high temperature, you may worry about the possibility of meningitis or septicaemia. Tables 1 and 2 give the main symptoms and signs of meningitis and of septicaemia caused by meningococcal bacteria. **Not everyone develops all these signs and symptoms. If your child is ill and you are worried, contact your doctor to ask for advice, saying that you are concerned about the possibility of meningitis. You may be reassured after talking to the doctor, or he/she may visit, or ask you to bring your child to the surgery or health centre, or even to go straight to hospital.**

Table 1. Meningitis and Septicaemia - what to look out for in babies under 1 to 2 years old:

General Signs of Infection
- high temperature
- vomiting
- no interest in feeding

Signs of possible Meningitis or Septicaemia
- unusual irritability
- moaning, high-pitched cry
- unusual drowsiness
- floppy
- body stiffening, or fits
- bulging soft spot on the top of the head
- cold, pale or blotchy skin
- red/purple spots, or bruises *(see The Glass Test - page 18)*

Table 2. Meningitis and Septicaemia - what to look out for in older children:

General Signs of Infection
- high temperature
- vomiting
- aches and pains in the joints and muscles.
- weakness

Signs of possible Meningitis or Septicaemia
- severe headache
- stiff neck
- dislike of bright light
- drowsiness or confusion
- fits
- cold, pale or blotchy skin
- red/purple spots or bruises. *(see The Glass Test - page18.)*

The "General Signs of Infection" listed at the top of each table (e.g. high temperature, vomiting) are regularly seen in other common illnesses like colds or the flu. When there is only high temperature and a runny nose, or diarrhoea and vomiting, meningitis is very unlikely. The reason for including these common symptoms and signs here is that they make up a part of the whole picture of meningitis. Colds are common, while meningitis is rare, and most children with general signs of infection do not have meningitis. Indeed,out of 10,000 children who have signs of a cold, an ear infection or flu, 9,999 will have just that and no more.

The "Signs of possible Meningitis or Septicaemia" - the second half of each table - should always be taken seriously. If any of these are seen, the general practitioner (GP) should be contacted without delay.

No-one should feel awkward about contacting the GP if worried about the possibility of such a serious illness, and they should mention their fear of meningitis. GPs are very anxious never to miss a case of serious illness like meningitis, and will always take the possibility very seriously.

Meningitis and Septicaemia in babies under one to two years old

Beyond the general signs of infection in a baby, such as a *high temperature* or *vomiting*, one of the first signs of meningitis, or of septicaemia caused by meningococcal bacteria, is often *irritability*, which may be marked by an unusual *moaning* or *high-pitched cry*. The baby may seem to dislike being touched, and it can be very difficult to comfort him/her in the usual ways. This is often combined with *unusual drowsiness*, even to the point of the baby being *difficult to wake up*. The baby may feel *floppy* to hold, and seem weak, only able to *suck poorly* at the breast or bottle.

One of the dangerous things that happens in meningitis is swelling of the brain. As a result, the *soft spot ("fontanelle")* on the top of the head may *bulge out* and feel hard. (When healthy babies cry, the soft spot often bulges out for a moment: this is quite normal, and nothing to worry about). Painful spasm of the neck muscles causes the classic sign of a *stiff neck* in meningitis, but this is often not seen in young babies, as the muscles are still weak. A baby with meningitis may have a *fit* (convulsion or seizure are other terms often used). In a fit the baby loses consciousness, the eyes appear to roll back, and the baby may stiffen or jerk his/her limbs.

What to do if someone has a fit

If your child goes into a fit, he/she should be laid in a safe place on his/her side with the head back, and the chin forward, so as to be sure that he/she can breathe safely. If the child is sick in this position, vomit should be cleaned quickly away from the mouth. The doctor should be contacted right away, and will usually arrange for urgent hospital admission in order to ensure that fits do not recur, and to find out the cause. Most fits in the 6 month to five year old age group turn out to be caused by a high temperature rather than by meningitis, but tests may be needed to rule out serious infection. Fits do not usually last longer than a few minutes. **If the fit does not stop quickly, and you cannot reach your doctor for help, you should call an ambulance.**

Although a baby with meningitis or septicaemia may have a high temperature, *the skin may feel cold* as the blood flow is diverted to internal organs. As a result, he/she may *look pale and blotchy*, or even *grey in colour*. In cases of meningitis or septicaemia caused by meningococcal bacteria, *red or purple spots, or bruises*, may appear. There may be only a few spots or marks, or a widespread rash. When there is a rash, not all the spots look the same. There may be a mixture of larger and smaller spots, some pink, others dark red, and some bruises. **There is more about these spots, which are important signs of septicaemia caused by meningococcal bacteria, on page 17, and pictures on pages 20-23.**

Meningitis and Septicaemia in toddlers, older children and adults.

In older children, as in babies, meningitis, or septicaemia caused by meningococcal bacteria, may develop in someone who until then has seemed entirely well, or may come on after a period of mild illness with a cold, earache or minor infection of that sort.

As before, the older child or adult with meningitis or septicaemia will usually have some general signs of infection: a *high temperature*, (which may be accompanied by *feeling cold or shivery*), or *vomiting*. *Aching joints or muscles* in the arms, legs or back, which can be very painful, are a common symptom of the flu but are also a feature of septicaemia caused by meningococcal bacteria. Other signs of meningitis and/or septicaemia caused by meningococcal bacteria are similar to those that have been described for babies and young children: *drowsiness* or *confusion*, *a fit*, *cold* and *pale* or *blotchy skin*, and most importantly, *red or purple spots or bruises* appearing on the skin. Making the diagnosis of meningitis in older children can be easier than it is in babies, as the child may be able to describe symptoms. An older child will often complain of *severe headache*. Some toddlers with only a few words may complain of *tummy ache* instead, though when asked to show where it hurts he/she may hold his/her head. A *stiff neck* is more commonly seen in older children than in babies, and can be checked by asking a child sitting in bed to kiss (or touch his/her forehead to) his/her knee. The spasm of the neck muscles that occurs in meningitis makes this painful or impossible. The child may complain that the *light hurts ("photophobia")*, or this may be obvious by the way that bright lights are avoided.

The spots seen in infections caused by meningococcal bacteria

In infections caused by meningococcal bacteria, spots are an important sign that dangerous infection of the blood (septicaemia) is developing. Although the spots are often described as a rash, this may be misleading. Sometimes instead of a widespread rash there are only a few tiny spots, or one or more bruises. They may first appear at sites where clothes have caused pressure on the skin - under elastic, for example. The spots may vary in size, and also in colour, from pink to dark red/purple (like a blood blister). The appearance and the number of the spots can change quickly, over an hour or two, as the illness progresses. **Pictures of the spots seen at different stages of infection caused by meningococcal bacteria are shown on plates 1 - 8, pages 20 - 23.**

Of course, many infections, mainly minor ones that get better without any specific treatment, are accompanied by rashes. Therefore the appearance of a rash in someone who is unwell does not automatically signify a very serious illness. However, the spots which may occur in infections caused by meningococcal bacteria differ in one particular respect from the spots seen in most other infections. Because they are formed by blood leaking out of tiny blood vessels into the surface layers of the skin, they do not fade on pressure. This can easily be checked at home using the **"glass test"**.

THE GLASS TEST.
illustrated with pictures on page 20.

Press the side of a drinking glass firmly against an area where there are spots and look through at the flattened skin. If there are quite a few spots, look at several different areas.

If any of the spots don't fade, then the glass test is positive. **See the picture on page 20.** The cause could be meningococcal septicaemia. **In this case you should contact a doctor immediately**.

If the pressure makes all the spots fade and lose colour then the test is negative. Fading spots are *NOT* typical of infection with meningococcal bacteria. You should check again after an hour or so, as in the earliest stages of infection the test may be negative, though it will become positive after a short time.

If the spots fade when you do the glass test but you are still worried, you should trust your instincts and get medical help in any case.

If you see just a few spots, or a whole rash of them, on your child's skin, do the glass test to check if they fade on pressure. If they do not fade, get medical help immediately, if necessary, by calling an ambulance. If the spots do fade on pressure, re-check after an hour or so to see if things have changed. In any case, if you are worried about your child, do not hesitate to contact your doctor for advice.

In some cases, rather than causing red spots, the leakage of blood into the surface layers of the skin causes the appearance of *bruising*. These may be anything from quite small bruises, to, occasionally, large bruised-looking areas of skin.

In any case of unexplained bruising, especially if it occurs in an ill person with a high temperature, get medical help immediately.

Further pictures of the sorts of spots and bruising seen in meningococcal sepsis are shown on pages 21 - 23.

The tables and text in this chapter - on the signs and symptoms of meningitis, and of septicaemia caused by meningococcal bacteria - provide detailed descriptions of the conditions to be sure that every aspect is covered. However, often only a few of the features are present, especially in the early stages. To make it easier to picture what an ill person with these conditions might really be like, the next chapter consists of true stories, written by patients or their parents, of their experiences.

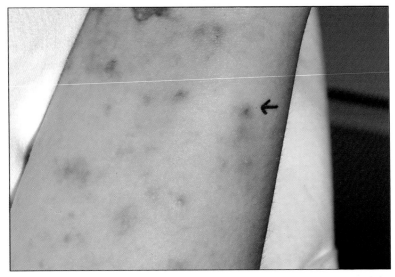

Plate 1. **The glass test** *(see page 18)*: Spots of meningococcal septicaemia.

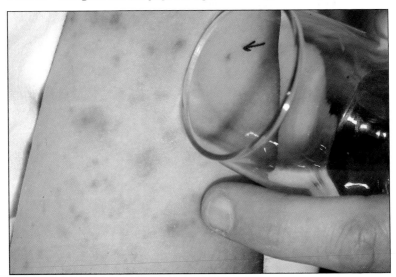

Plate 2. **The glass test** *(see page 18)*: The same spots with a glass pressed on them. Some spots have faded, but one (arrowed) remains. The test is POSITIVE.

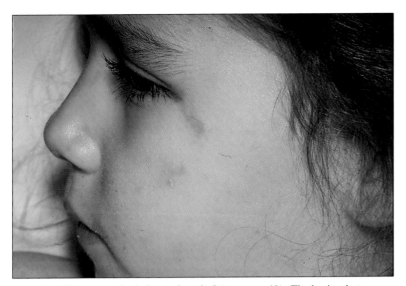

Plate 3. **Noora on admission to hospital** *(see page 41)*. The bruise that suddenly appeared under her eye.

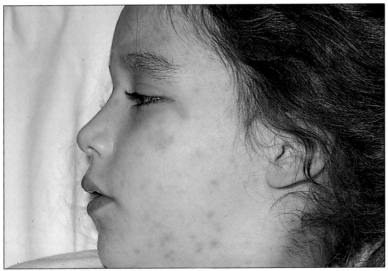

Plate 4. **Noora's face a little later** *(see page 41)*. More spots quickly appeared.

Plate 5. **Spots of early septicaemia caused by meningococcal bacteria.** Sometimes there can be very few, small spots in this serious illness, as seen on this child's chest.

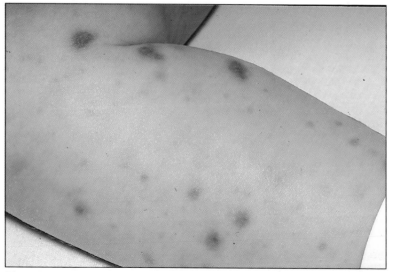

Plate 6. **Spots of meningococcal septicaemia.** Larger, more obvious spots on this baby's leg.

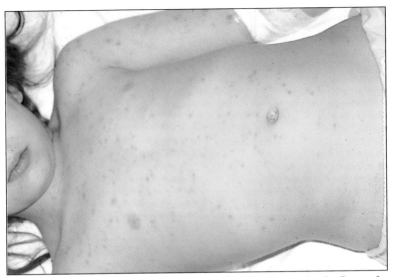

Plate 7.   Spots in meningococcal septicaemia. A widespread rash. Some of the spots faded under pressure (the glass test) but others did not.

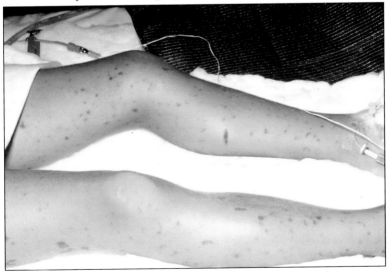

Plate 8.   Spots of meningococcal septicaemia. A widespread rash of spots nearly all of which remained (did not fade) when the glass test was carried out.

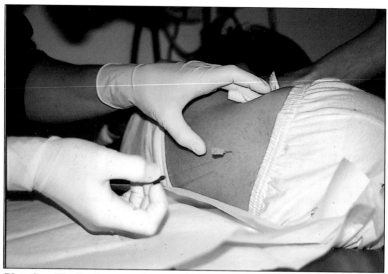

Plate 9. **The lumbar puncture test** *(see page 76).* Cerebrospinal fluid is dripping out of the needle that can be seen in the child's back.

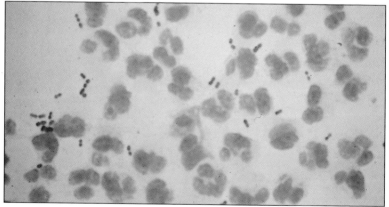

Plate 10. **Cerebrospinal fluid containing pneumococcal bacteria and human white blood cells, from a case of meningitis.** A sample of fluid has been placed on a microscope slide and treated with a stain to show up any cells and bacteria. This is its appearance down the microscope. The large red-brown stained objects are white blood cells which have entered the cerebrospinal fluid to fight the infection. The small blue-black stained objects are pneumococcal bacteria that have caused this child's meningitis.

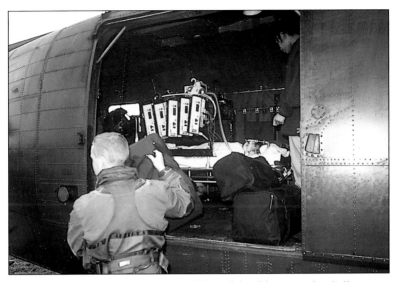

Plate 11. Emergency transport. A child receiving life support in a helicopter on the way to the children's intensive care unit.

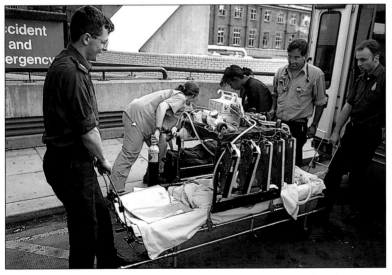

Plate 12. Emergency transport. A child on life support is transferred to an ambulance.

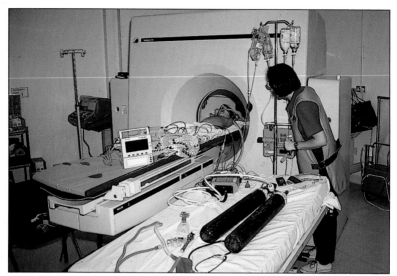

Plate 13.   The CT scanner *(see page 78)*. The child's head is almost invisible in the machine. The X-rays are taken from within the large ring (that looks like a washing machine door).

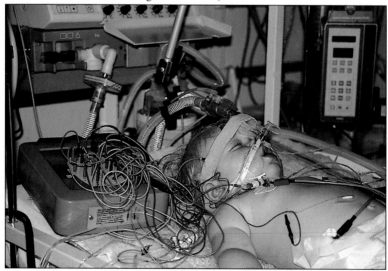

Plate 14.   An EEG test *(see page 79)*. Electrodes are stuck to the child's head with sticky gel so that the brain waves can be recorded.

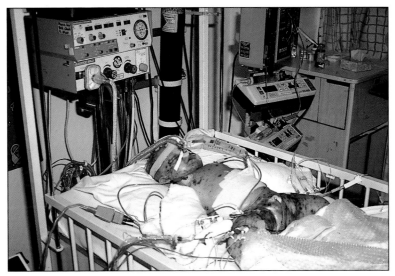

Plate 15. **Child with meningococcal septicaemia.** Desperately ill on the intensive care unit.

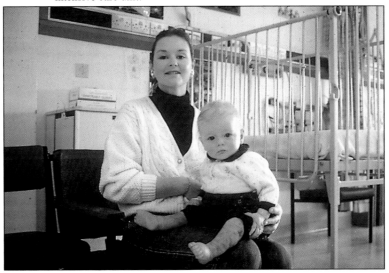

Plate 16. **Triumph!** The same child as shown in plate 15. He has made a complete recovery, except for extensive scarring of his legs caused by the disease.

CHAPTER 2
Case histories

Introduction

The signs and symptoms of meningitis, and of septicaemia caused by meningococcal bacteria, were described in the last chapter. To illustrate how these illnesses appear in real life, this chapter contains twelve true stories, most of them written by the parents of patients, but some by the patients themselves. Each account ends at around the time that the patient reached hospital, and is followed by a commentary picking up the key points, referring back each time to features of meningitis or septicaemia described in Chapter 1. At the end of each commentary there is a check list of signs and symptoms, laid out like table 1 or 2 in the last chapter.

These accounts give a realistic picture of what happens as someone falls ill with meningitis, or with septicaemia caused by meningococcal bacteria. They help to show the differences between someone with a mild infection that is going to get better on its own and someone who is developing a life-threatening illness. These differences can seem subtle when put into words, so it is important to keep things sensibly in perspective. Meningitis, and septicaemia caused by meningococcal bacteria, are rare diseases. Thousands of children will have minor illnesses for each one that has meningitis or septicaemia. However, in each of the cases described, the reader can see that the illness progressed to something that was clearly out of the ordinary. Early on there may have been nothing to distinguish each case from one of minor illness, and where doctors were involved at these earliest stages, they were not wrong to be reassuring. However, in most cases the parents were asked to contact the doctor again if there were any changes or new worries. These are never empty words, and the stories make it very clear how important it is to keep vigilant with a sick child, checking on him/her regularly, including during the night, and not to hold back from contacting the doctor again if the picture should change.

One of the mysteries about meningococcal disease is the great variation that is seen in the rate with which victims fall ill. One child may have an illness which develops slowly, over a day or two. Another may be desperately ill within hours of the first hint that anything is wrong. This is described vividly in some of these stories. It is cases like these that prompted us to write this book. We wanted to do the best we could to be sure that parents knew when they should get a doctor to see their sick children, and that older people recognised when they themselves might need a doctor urgently.

Names, places and dates have been changed.

Jamie, aged 2. His father's story

6 am: it seemed to be a normal start to a normal day. I was getting up for work and the boys were awake, but the smallest, Jamie, seemed a bit under the weather. My wife said he was very warm and docile. He lay in our bed, sleeping for 5-10 minutes at a time, then waking. He'd done this for about 2 hours. He seemed very hot. I took his temp: just over 100°F (38°C). Another half hour and I took it again, this time nearly 104°F (40°C). He seemed agitated (didn't like being touched) so we rang the Emergency Doctor, described the symptoms and he came. He said Jamie's drowsiness was probably down to his temperature. He said he didn't think it was meningitis because Jamie's neck wasn't stiff, but he couldn't find a reason why he should be so hot: it may be a urine infection, he said. He told us he would get another doctor to call after surgery to check Jamie's condition. About 9.00 he left, and Jamie fell back to sleep. He woke about half-an-hour later very drowsy but asking for a drink. We gave him one but within minutes he was vomiting: then he fell back to sleep. We were getting worried: Jamie had never been sick before. What was also strange was that he had not asked for any breakfast. He awoke again at about 10.30 asking for another drink, and again as soon as it was down he brought it up. With this my wife rang the surgery again. They said the doctor would be around straight away after morning surgery - we would be the first call. But in the meantime could we get a urine sample ready for when the Doc came. I tried to get Jamie to stand up for a wee but he couldn't. He was so weak, his little legs couldn't support him. His energy seemed to be nearly all gone. He couldn't hardly cry even. At 11.00 I took his temp again now it was nearly 105°F (41°C). I took his pyjamas off and noticed a little red blotch at the top of his leg. It looked like a little love-bite or pinch. My wife noticed another on his belly. At 11.30 the doctor came. She looked him over and there were more blotches or little spots appearing all over his body. Right away she rang the ambulance. By 12.00 he was on the critical list at the local hospital.

Comment

Jamie had septicaemia caused by meningococcal bacteria. He did not have meningitis. He needed life support on the intensive care unit for one day, but went on to make a complete recovery.

When Jamie was first seen by the doctor there was nothing obviously serious about his illness. A child with a high temperature, who is very sleepy and irritable ("didn't like being touched") unquestionably needs to be seen by a doctor: among other things it could be meningitis or septicaemia. However, Jamie seemed quite a bit better when the doctor came round. Some children, like Amy in the next story, and Lily *(see page 47)*, have brief periods of seeming pretty much alright even though the illness is progressing. Jamie's doctor thought of meningitis and checked, but Jamie's neck wasn't stiff. (In meningococcal septicaemia without meningitis, however, there is no neck stiffness). Although he could not make a diagnosis and thought that probably nothing serious was wrong, he wanted another doctor to see him again later in the morning. Doctors will often do this, as they know that children can change for the worse very quickly. The diagnosis may be much easier to make with new signs showing after just a few hours, and the right treatment can then be started. It is important though that parents do not feel that such an arrangement means that they cannot contact the doctor sooner - as Jamie's story shows. Within a couple of hours he was clearly worse - very drowsy and weak, and vomiting - and his mother contacted the doctor again, just in time. By the time the GP arrived an hour later, the spots of septicaemia caused by meningococcal bacteria were beginning to appear. A "love-bite or pinch" is a very good description of what the spots can sometimes look like. If Jamie had not got to hospital soon afterwards, the illness might have been much more serious or even fatal.

The table adjacent is a reminder of the features of meningitis and septicaemia caused by meningococcal bacteria. The ticks mark Jamie's symptoms and signs.

Jamie, aged 2	
High temperature	✔
Vomiting	✔
Pains in muscles and joints	
Weakness	✔
Severe headache	
Stiff neck	
Dislikes bright lights	
Drowsy or Confused	✔
Fits	
Cold/pale/blotchy skin	
Red/purple spots or bruises	✔

Amy, aged 14. Her own story

I had a normal day at school on Wednesday, although I'd had a cold since the weekend. That evening a shooting pain developed in the upper part of my back. I went to bed early, but I was awake a lot during the night with bad pains in my back and legs. In the morning I had a high temperature, and it was obvious I couldn't go to school. My Dad stayed at home with me, and when my Mum came home at lunch time, I was lying in bed with a temperature and a sore throat, feeling slightly sick. We noticed a pink blotchy rash on my arms and legs, but it disappeared as my temperature went down after paracetamol. My Mum said she thought I had a nasty virus.

Around 6 o'clock I felt a bit better and had a bath, but when I got out I felt very dizzy and fainted. I was helped downstairs, where I sat on the sofa speaking to my friend on the phone. When I'd finished on the phone, a very bad headache developed quickly. I've often had headaches, but nowhere near as painful as this one. I went back to bed with some aspirin. The headache didn't get any better, and I remember being sick, but nothing else until I woke up in hospital a week later.

Amy, aged 14. Her mother's story

We had been worried that Amy's headache seemed so bad, and that she'd been sick, but we felt reassured because the high fever that she'd had earlier in the day had gone, and that as the evening wore on she stopped crying with the head pain and seemed to be drifting off to sleep. She was more comfortable without the light on, so we sat with her in the dark. I left the room for a few minutes, and when I returned, I found that she had vomited again. I started to talk to her, and suddenly realised that she wasn't responding to me normally, and didn't realise what was happening. I turned on the light and saw that she was very pale and felt very cold.

After this we became very frightened and rang the hospital to tell them we were rushing Amy in. Then we had difficulty getting Amy downstairs and into the car - she couldn't support her weight and was only half conscious. She seemed to get worse on the 20 minute journey. She seemed to be slipping from us. We lifted her into a wheelchair and ran along darkened hospital corridors to the treatment room on the children's ward. In its bright lights we saw for the first time a purple-red rash appearing on her body and legs.

Comment

Amy had meningitis and septicaemia caused by meningococcal bacteria, and nearly died. She was unconscious by the time she reached hospital, was transferred to a specialist children's intensive care unit and remained in a coma on life support for a week before coming round. There were fears that she had suffered some brain damage as she had a squint and double vision for a while, but fortunately she got completely back to normal after a month.

From her high temperature and aches and pains at the start of her illness, Amy could simply have had flu or some other harmless virus infection. Her parents thought that this was the likely diagnosis and felt comfortable looking after her at home as her father is a doctor. It was later that the very worrying symptoms developed: splitting headache (the worst Amy had ever had), dislike of the light, vomiting, and then drowsiness, confusion, and the paleness and coldness.

Amy was able to chat to her friend on the telephone even though only a short time before she had felt terrible and had fainted. Children with meningococcal septicaemia may sometimes struggle on, and for brief periods even seem not to be all that ill, until the infection is quite advanced (for other examples, see Jamie's and Lily's stories *(pages 29 and 47)*. This should never put parents off contacting the doctor if they are worried about their child.

The table adjacent is a reminder of the features of meningitis and septicaemia caused by meningococcal bacteria. The ticks mark Amy's symptoms and signs.

Amy, aged 14	
High temperature	✔
Vomiting	✔
Pains in muscles and joints	✔
Weakness	✔
Severe headache	✔
Stiff neck	
Dislikes bright lights	✔
Drowsy or Confused	✔
Fits	
Cold/pale/blotchy skin	✔
Red/purple spots or bruises	✔

Grace, aged 3. Her father's story

When I collected Grace from her child minder I was told that she'd had a temperature that afternoon but that it had come down with paracetamol. This was no real surprise as she'd had a cough and runny nose for over a week, though she hadn't seemed ill with it. Around 9.00 pm her temperature rose again so we gave her more paracetamol. She didn't seem right - she was hot, breathing shallowly, and she said her hands ached so she didn't want to suck her fingers to help her sleep. We decided to call the doctor. When he came he felt Grace probably had bronchitis, and prescribed some medicine. After taking the medicine Grace was sick and when we changed her pyjamas we found spots on her body. The books we have at home made us think of a virus like measles, especially as she'd had watery eyes a few days earlier. We phoned the doctor again and he agreed that it could be measles and that the medication was the same.

All that night Grace had a very high temperature, which we tried to control with wet cloths and a fan.

In the morning my wife went off to work, leaving me to phone the doctor once the surgery was open to confirm that Grace's illness was going as we should expect. I felt this was unnecessary, but my wife is usually right in these things.

When I gave Grace her medicine she was sick again. Then she began to look awful. She was flat out on the bed with pale lips and an ashen face, but she didn't feel hot to touch any more. Our GP came round soon after, and as soon as she saw Grace she got very worried. She was more interested in the spots than anything else. She said it didn't look like measles, and that we should go to the hospital straight away, as she was worried that it might be meningitis. When she said the M word I was on the phone in a flash. I called 4 cab firms and our child minder to take us. Meanwhile the doctor gave Grace an injection of penicillin. Grace was completely still like a rag doll in my arms, and she only whimpered when the needle went in: usually she would have screamed the place down. By now there was a queue of taxis waiting outside. I jumped into the nearest one with Grace, and we rushed to the hospital. Our GP had phoned ahead, and the team of doctors and nurses were ready to go to work on us as soon as we arrived.

Comment

Grace had septicaemia caused by meningococcal bacteria. Shortly after she reached her local hospital she got so much worse that she needed life support. She was collected from her local hospital by a specialised team of doctors and taken by ambulance to a children's intensive care unit. She responded well to treatment and made a complete recovery.

The signs that Grace had something more serious than bronchitis only appeared on the second day of her illness. Her fever, sickness, aching hands and rash could have been caused by any number of mild virus infections, and did not point definitely to a serious infection. The things that made her parents realise that they needed the doctor again urgently were her extreme floppiness, pale colour, cold skin - signs in fact that the bacteria were spreading through her bloodstream and she had septicaemia. The rash that appeared the evening before might have been a warning sign. People often put a child's rash down to "measles" but in fact this is now rare thanks to the measles, mumps and rubella (MMR) vaccine (see chapter 8). Any floppy, sick child with high fever and a rash should be seen by a doctor. **If spots appear on your child after the doctor has been, you should not feel**

awkward about contacting the doctor again. The most likely thing is still that the cause is a minor infection, but the possibility of dangerous, rapidly advancing disease caused by meningococcal bacteria needs to be considered.

When the doctor came the second time she was very worried that Grace might have an infection with meningococcal bacteria, and this is why she gave he ran injection of penicillin antibiotic straight away. All GPs carry this with them in their bags for just this sort of emergency. This injection and, even more important, the instinct that Grace's mother felt in getting the doctor to see her again even before she seemed really bad, may well have saved her life.

The table adjacent is a reminder of the features of meningitis and septicaemia caused by meningococcal bacteria. The ticks mark Grace's symptoms and signs.

Grace, aged 3	
High temperature	✔
Vomiting	✔
Pains in muscles and joints	✔
Weakness	✔
Severe headache	
Stiff neck	
Dislikes bright lights	
Drowsy or Confused	✔
Fits	
Cold/pale/blotchy skin	✔
Red/purple spots or bruises	✔

Hawra, aged 3. Her mother's story

Until Saturday night there was nothing wrong at all with Hawra. All that day she was completely normal, active and playing around and her usual self.

She went to sleep at 9.00 pm. Half an hour later I heard strange sounds coming from her bedroom. I rushed up and found her freezing cold and shivering, so I put a couple of blankets over her. She was shivering on and off for about an hour, then suddenly she became very hot and had a fit. Hawra had never had a fit before and I was very frightened but my husband said "children get fits because of high temperature", so we started to put ice on her forehead and her feet. It seemed to help a little bit but she was still very hot. Her temperature was 104°F (40°C), she was talking nonsense all night and complaining of having a headache.

At midnight she vomited once, and at 7.00 in the morning she had another fit, so we called the ambulance. They came straight away and rushed us to the hospital. The doctors noticed a rash of tiny pink-red spots on her skin, and said they thought she had meningococcal septicaemia.

Comment

Hawra had meningitis and septicaemia caused by meningococcal bacteria. She spent five days in the intensive care unit, three of them on life support, and a further week in hospital before making a complete recovery.

The first sign that Hawra was ill was her violent shivering. This is usually a sign that a child is developing a high temperature. The hands and feet often feel very cold as the blood circulation of the skin is cut right down to stop heat being lost and so build up the temperature more quickly. Some children can have fits with high temperatures *(see box, page 15)* - something which can run in families. If parents are used to dealing with their children's fits with high temperatures they may not even contact the doctor, but you should *always* do so if your child has not had a fit before or if you are at all worried. Sometimes a fit can be a sign of a serious illness affecting the brain, like meningitis.

Through the night Hawra's illness got worse. The high temperature, second fit, confusion ("talking nonsense") and headache all point to the possibility of meningitis. Luckily her parents got her to hospital just in time.

The table adjacent is a reminder of the features of meningitis and septicaemia caused by meningococcal bacteria. The ticks mark Hawra's symptoms and signs.

Hawra, aged 3	
High temperature	✔
Vomiting	✔
Pains in muscles and joints	
Weakness	
Severe headache	✔
Stiff neck	
Dislikes bright lights	
Drowsy or Confused	✔
Fits	✔
Cold/pale/blotchy skin	
Red/purple spots or bruises	✔

Sam, aged 8 months. His mother's story

The first signs of Sam's illness were very minor and began two days before we became really concerned about him. On the first day he gradually became more and more irritable and, unusually for him, began to refuse some of his feeds. He didn't sleep through the night either but as he was teething quite badly we put this down to sore gums and hunger.

The next day, he slept much more than usual (which we had half expected following such a broken night), but between sleeps he seemed to be his normal bright, alert and happy self. He had another broken night, waking up and crying as if he was in pain, but again we put this down to teething, and teething gel seemed to settle him.

On the third day he woke much later than usual and was clearly unwell - miserable, moaning quietly, hot, pale and not really interested in any of his toys or his food. He also flopped over when we tried to sit him up and seemed to prefer just lying down without moving and going to sleep. We called the GP who found that his temperature was 102°F (39°C) and that one of his ear drums was pink. He'd had an ear infection ten days previously which had settled very quickly with antibiotics and she wondered whether this was recurring. She prescribed more antibiotics and paracetamol, and advised us to call again if he didn't improve fairly quickly.

Sam spent most of that afternoon asleep and when we woke him to give his antibiotic he was clearly worse - still very hot in spite of paracetamol, even more drowsy, pale, and floppy - and we noticed that the soft spot on the top of his head was beginning to bulge. Every now and then he would arch his back and neck and cry out and then lie completely still again. He was completely uninterested in everything - we wondered if he even recognised us - and only responded to being picked up, when he would cry as if he was in pain. We gave him his medicine and offered him some of his favourite yogurt but it just made him violently sick.

By now we were very worried and quite frightened and asked the doctor to come again urgently. She came within half an hour but even in that short time he'd got worse. She wasn't sure exactly what was wrong so she advised us to take him straight to hospital and contacted the doctors there to tell them to expect us. On the journey he continued to get more and more sleepy and floppy and was violently sick again just after we arrived. Thankfully the diagnosis of meningitis was made very quickly when the doctors did a lumbar puncture, and he was started on treatment straight away.

Comment

Sam had meningitis caused by pneumococcal bacteria. He was in hospital on treatment for nearly two weeks and made a full recovery.

Pneumococcal bacteria are responsible for about one in five cases of meningitis that are caused by bacteria. The germ is a common cause of ear infections, and cases of meningitis may follow an earlier ear infection. Of course nearly all such ear infections clear up completely with a course of antibiotic medicine. Meningitis is a very rare complication, but the story that Sam's mother tells is typical of the occasions when it does occur.

At the start of his illness, Sam's parents thought he was just teething. At this stage the bacteria were probably just beginning to invade his body, but there were no signs to point to what was happening. However, when he developed a high temperature and was pale, uninterested in his food or his toys, and just moaning and sleepy, his mother (who is a doctor herself) got anxious for the GP to see him. It seemed that Sam's earlier ear infection might be coming back, but the doctor was worried in case there might be a more serious infection and warned Sam's parents to call her back if he should not get better quickly with the new medicine. Children's illnesses can get better very quickly but they can also get worse quickly, and parents must feel quite comfortable about calling the doctor back even after a very short time if they are worried. Sam did quickly get worse. Over the next few hours he developed many signs of meningitis. He got even more drowsy, pale, floppy, arching his back, vomiting, irritable (crying if picked up), and not recognising his parents. The soft spot at the top of his head was bulging out, a sign of the brain swelling that goes with meningitis. His parents quickly got the doctor back, Sam was sent to hospital as an emergency, and life-saving treatment was started soon after.

The table adjacent is a reminder of the features of meningitis. The ticks mark Sam's symptoms and signs.

Sam, aged 8 months	
High temperature	✔
Vomiting	✔
Uninterested in feeding	✔
Irritable	✔
Moaning/high-pitched cry	✔
Drowsy	✔
Floppy	✔
Stiffening/fits	
Bulging soft spot on head	✔
Cold/pale/blotchy skin	✔
Red/purple spots or bruises	

Edward, aged 15 months. His mother's story

Edward was 15 months old and teething. On Tuesday evening he was niggly, and that night he didn't sleep very well. Wednesday dawned and he seemed bright enough so we got through the day without too many worries, but again he slept poorly. On Thursday he slept most of the time, but I wasn't too worried as I thought he was catching up from the previous two nights. He showed no signs of being uncomfortable, or hot, and he was not crying, but he just drifted in and out of sleep, not interested in anything.

That evening I was due to go out to band practice, and I did just wonder with my husband if we should ring the doctor, but we agreed not to as Edward showed no signs of being ill, just tired, and he was easily wakeable. As band practice finished I was just packing up and chatting when my husband burst in saying we had to get Edward to hospital right away. He had called the doctor as Edward had had a funny turn - his eyes, as he put it, had rolled up into his head - and that he'd been very difficult to rouse. The doctor had said he wasn't sure what was wrong but it could be serious, and that we should get him to hospital straight away. We rushed home in a blind panic, and packed a limp, very pale looking Edward into the car with our other son Andrew and set off on the 12 mile drive to hospital. Luckily we knew the way as the previous year we'd had to take Andrew in with what was eventually diagnosed as septic arthritis in his ankle. In hospital we spent a while going over what had happened, and how Edward had been over the last few days. Though he didn't have a high temperature and there were no obvious signs of infection they decided to do a "septic screen" to search everywhere for a cause, and that included a lumbar puncture to check for meningitis. We left the room while it was done, and when the doctor came out he said that the fluid was a little cloudy, a sign that it could be meningitis. Edward was transferred to the high dependency unit and treatment was started right away.

Comment

Like Sam in the previous story, Edward had meningitis caused by pneumococcal bacteria, but his illness was much more severe. He was unconscious for three days in the high dependency unit, and after he came round he was found to have become deaf as a result of the infection. This complication is seen more often with meningitis caused by pneumococcal bacteria than in other varieties of the disease. The coincidence of both Edward and his brother Andrew having severe infections led to many tests being done, resulting in the discovery that both boys had a deficiency in their immune systems making them particularly vulnerable. They are both now on regular treatment to prevent further problems. *How Edward's hearing problems were managed is described on page 87 in chapter 5 (What happens after Meningitis?).*

Edward's illness, like Sam's in the previous story, did not seem at all serious at the start. It is easy to be wise after the event and point to his drowsiness and lack of interest in things on the day he got worse, but of course many children who are teething and have had two unsettled nights can be just like that. The first sign that anything serious was wrong came when he had a"funny turn", which was probably a fit *(see box, page 15)*. When babies have fits their limbs and bodies often do not jerk very obviously. They may just go stiff briefly, their eyes "roll up into their heads", and they are then very drowsy for a while. Rushing Edward to hospital must have been life saving. Even in hospital it was not obvious what was wrong. The signs of meningitis can be very hard to see, especially in babies. Doctors will often do a whole lot of tests to find out where the infection is in an ill baby of Edward's age (a "septic screen"), and powerful antibiotic treatment will usually be started even before any answers have come back from the hospital laboratory.

The table adjacent is a reminder of the features of meningitis. The ticks mark Edward's symptoms and signs.

Edward, aged 15 months	
High temperature	
Vomiting	
Uninterested in feeding	
Irritable	
Moaning/high-pitched cry	
Drowsy	✔
Floppy	✔
Stiffening/fits	✔
Bulging soft spot on head	
Cold/pale/blotchy skin	✔
Red/purple spots or bruises	

Noora, aged 6. Her mother's story

On Saturday morning Noora attended Arabic School as usual, but that afternoon she had two bouts of diarrhoea. Sunday, she and her two sisters played quite happily, and there didn't seem to be any further problem. However, on Monday morning, while I was helping her dress for school, she seemed to be terribly tired. She rested on the sofa for a while, and I thought her colour looked odd: her complexion was a greyish colour. She was obviously sickening for something - perhaps the diarrhoea was going to come back - so I decided to keep her home from school. After a little she developed a fever so I gave her paracetamol. She said she felt hungry and I gave her some breakfast, but she quickly vomited so I just gave her some clear fluids. Again she vomited, and again I gave her just a drink of water, though she said she wanted something to eat. Through the morning she became more and more lethargic, with a high fever (104°F (40°C)) which wasn't coming down much with paracetamol. I couldn't get her to the toilet so I brought a potty to her. Then I noticed a bruise on her left cheek, below her eye, and found a rash beginning to develop all over her body. At the same time she started to complain of pains in her joints. I was now very worried about her and called the doctor immediately. He came within a short time, and immediately sent us to the hospital, phoning ahead to warn them that we were on our way.

Comment

Noora had septicaemia caused by meningococcal bacteria, but she did not have meningitis. Shortly after arriving in hospital her rash got much more widespread, as the septicaemia developed. However, she never needed life support, and after a week was well on the way to a complete recovery. The things that made her mother contact the emergency doctor are all things seen when this serious illness begins to take a hold: high fever, vomiting, not wanting to do anything except curl up and sleep (lethargy), pains in the joints, and in particular the bruises and other spots that began to appear (Noora's first bruise and later rash is shown in plates 3 and 4, page 21). It was the careful watch that her mother kept on Noora that led to her seeing the change in her daughter's condition and the new signs, making her get help at once and saving her daughter's life.

The table adjacent is a reminder of the features of meningitis and septicaemia caused by meningococcal bacteria. The ticks mark Noora's symptoms and signs.

Noora, aged 6	
High temperature	✔
Vomiting	✔
Pains in muscles and joints	✔
Weakness	
Severe headache	
Stiff neck	
Dislikes bright lights	
Drowsy or Confused	✔
Fits	
Cold/pale/blotchy skin	✔
Red/purple spots or bruises	✔

Antonia, aged 21. Her mother's story

Three days after Christmas, my daughter and I drove down from Bromsgrove to Taunton to visit relatives for a couple of days.

We had a lovely afternoon playing with my grandson, and that evening, by a strange coincidence, we talked about meningitis, as my daughter-in-law had memorised the symptoms from a poster on the baby clinic wall. At 11.30, as we went to bed, Toni complained that her shoulder was hurting - she thought she may have been sitting awkwardly on a bean bag.

At 3.30 in the morning Toni woke up and was violently sick. She complained of a bad headache, and I noticed a blood-blister on her eye-lid. She took some pain-killers and tried to get back to sleep, but tossed and turned for the rest of the night. The next morning we all assumed she had flu or some other virus, with a severe headache, aching joints, and a slight temperature. She had in fact just got over a sore throat, and just about everyone we knew had those sorts of symptoms. We decided that we should get back home as soon as possible. I thought Toni would be more comfortable at home, and I was worried in case I fell ill too and we both needed looking after. After our conversation of the night before meningitis crossed our minds, but it seemed ridiculous to contemplate such a coincidence! Nevertheless, just to be on the safe side, we looked for a rash. We didn't really know what we were looking for (but we did know that if we

*found any spots we had to press a glass over them to see if they went away).
Toni looked down her front and I looked at her back: nothing there. We
laughed at ourselves for being so silly!*

*Toni dozed for most of the drive home. When we stopped at a service
station Toni seemed very unsteady on her feet, but I put that down to her
having been asleep.*

*We got home at last around tea-time, and Toni staggered into the house
and flopped on to the settee. I took her temperature and it was below normal.
My husband had a virus just before Christmas and he had a low temperature
then, so we thought Toni must have the same bug. We discussed calling the
doctor but Toni went to sleep again so we decided to wait until she woke up
to see how she was then.*

*At 7 o'clock Toni woke up and was sick all over herself. As I helped her
take off her soiled jumper she asked "What are all these bruises on my
arm?" I literally ran to the telephone. Our GP was brilliant. I listed my
daughter's symptoms and she asked "Are the spots like bruises or blood
blisters?". I answered "Yes, actually they are just like small love-bites", and
I told her about the blood-blister on Toni's eye-lid. She asked us to bring
Toni straight round to the surgery, and met us at the door. She examined
Toni very quickly, and injected a large dose of Penicillin. She had already
called the hospital to check if there was a bed in the intensive care unit, and
we set of whilst she telephoned to confirm that we were on our way. As we
arrived, to be met at the door of the hospital by a nurse with a wheel-chair,
Toni was covered all over with bruises, and her hands were so very very
cold.*

Comment

Antonia had septicaemia caused by meningococcal bacteria. She was cared
for in the intensive care unit for four days before going to a regular hospital
ward, where she stayed for two weeks. Very fortunately she made a complete
recovery.

In the early stages of Antonia's illness, as described in so many of the other stories here, there was nothing to mark it out as special. It was the time of year that everyone was getting virus infections like flu, as her father had done. The pain in her shoulder and later the joint pains, the headache, the slight temperature - these are all common complaints that usually get better with no more than some paracetamol, comforting hot drinks and a day or two of rest. One of the most difficult things for patients, their parents or doctors to do is to recognise a case of severe illness - as Antonia's was to become - when there are lots of cases of mild illness about. Therefore it is worth stressing the things that rang the alarm bells in Antonia's case.

First the spots. Antonia and her mother knew that "a rash" could be a sign of "meningitis" - actually, this is a sign that meningococcal bacteria are infecting the bloodstream, causing septicaemia - and they knew about the "glass test" *(see box, page 18, and plates 1 and 2, page 20)* but they did not know exactly what these spots were supposed to look like. As plates 1 - 8 on pages 20 - 23 and the stories in this book make clear, they can be very varied. They can be little dark red spots like a blood blister, or bigger marks, like "love bites" (as in Antonia herself and as described in Jamie's story *page 29*). They can look like bruises (as in Noora's story *page 41*). Different sorts of spots may appear at different stages, and they can change in appearance in the space of just one or two hours. It is really better not to think of the spots as a "rash", as most people then picture lots of spots all over the body, not just one or two spots, marks or bruises - but this is all that may be seen. The glass test, described in the box on page 18, with pictures on page 20, can be used to check if spots disappear or remain visible when the skin is pressed. If they remain visible, this is a sign that they are caused by bleeding into the skin. You should contact the doctor straight away if you find these spots on yourself or your sick child.

Next the drowsiness. Drowsiness with a fever can be a sign of serious infection. Although tiredness on its own is of course nothing unusual, especially after a disturbed night, a doctor should be consulted about any one of any age with a high temperature who seems at all hard to wake up.

Finally, the feeling of coldness. All the publicity about meningitis stresses the high temperature, so the idea of coldness being a sign of the illness may seem odd. There are two reasons why someone with an infection may feel cold to the touch. If someone is developing a high temperature, the hands and feet in particular may feel cold as the body is conserving heat as hard as it can by diverting the blood flow away from the skin. The temperature taken with a thermometer under the tongue is usually high in these cases. This was described in Hawra's story *(page 35)*. However, pale, cold skin is a regular feature of the very serious illness of meningococcal septicaemia. The victim may feel very cold to the touch as the circulation is no longer working properly and the blood flow to the skin is cut right down to keep up the supply to vital internal organs.

The table adjacent is a reminder of the features of meningitis and septicaemia caused by meningococcal bacteria. The ticks mark Antonia's symptoms and signs.

Antonia, aged 21	
High temperature	✔
Vomiting	✔
Pains in muscles and joints	✔
Weakness	✔
Severe headache	✔
Stiff neck	
Dislikes bright lights	
Drowsy or Confused	✔
Fits	
Cold/pale/blotchy skin	✔
Red/purple spots or bruises	✔

Amanda, aged 20. Her own story

On Saturday I woke up with a muzzy head and sore throat, but I didn't think anything of it at first. My friend picked me up at 11 am and I suggested we go for an ice cream before work, to soothe my throat. By lunch time I was feeling lousy. My head was pounding and I felt cold, so much so that I had to put my jacket on, even though it was the middle of June. It was then that my friend pointed out that my lips had turned blue. I decided to go back to my student flat where I packed up some things and drove to my parents home. They were away visiting friends, but I explained to the neighbours that I thought I had flu, let myself in, locked the door and headed straight for bed.

Next time I woke it was Sunday and things went from bad to worse. I began to feel very vague and distant. My headache was now unbearable and my neck was aching. I hardly had the strength to crawl to the bathroom with sickness and diarrhoea. I became aware of purply-blue blotches on my skin and I now realised I had to get help. Luckily I had a phone at my bedside because by now I was so weak I could not find the energy to get up. I tried to contact my parents but they were out and it was some time later that I managed to get hold of my mum and explained the situation. She was horrified. She immediately contacted my GP, my uncle and a neighbour. My uncle was the last person I can remember seeing that day. Being security conscious I had double locked the front door and left the key in the lock, and my neighbour and uncle had to knock the door down to get to me.

Comment

Amanda had meningitis and septicaemia caused by meningococcal bacteria. She was still conscious and able to talk to the doctor when he arrived, though she remembers nothing of that. She was rushed to hospital and by two hours later she was so ill that her heart stopped beating. She was resuscitated and survived after nine days on life support in intensive care, though she was left with brain damage. *You can read the rest of her story on page 85 in chapter 5 (What happens after Meningitis?).*

When Amanda's illness started, things like her sore throat, the muzzy, lousy, feeling she described and her pounding headache could all have been caused by a virus infection like the flu, though this is quite unusual in the summer months. Quickly, though, it got far worse than any common infection, and if anyone had been with her they would surely have called a doctor urgently. The rapid way in which her illness worsened, with vomiting and diarrhoea, the unbearable headache and neck ache, the confusion ("vague feeling"), the weakness and the purple rash are all features of meningitis and septicaemia caused by meningococcal bacteria. It is very lucky that Amanda had the sense and strength to make that phone call for help: in a very few hours she would almost certainly have died. **If you live on your own it is a**

Amanda, aged 20	
High temperature	✔
Vomiting	✔
Pains in muscles and joints	
Weakness	✔
Severe headache	✔
Stiff neck	✔
Dislikes bright lights	
Drowsy or Confused	✔
Fits	
Cold/pale/blotchy skin	✔
Red/purple spots or bruises	✔

good idea to tell someone if you are feeling ill, and ask them to ring or call round to check how you are doing.

The table above is a reminder of the features of meningitis and septicaemia caused by meningococcal bacteria. The ticks mark Amanda's symptoms and signs.

Lily, aged 3. Her mother's story

On Sunday morning, after a disturbed night, Lily seemed tired and uninterested in things. As I took her pyjamas off to wash her, I noticed she had a rash. I thought it must be the start of chicken pox, as it was going round and she hadn't had it, so I assumed that it was now our turn. Lily ate a little breakfast, but vomited later. She didn't want her lunch, and was quite groggy, very quiet and lying still, not interested in anything. I was concerned about this - Lily had not been ill before, so I didn't know what to expect.

After lunch I phoned the doctor. Because it was a Sunday I had been going to wait until the next morning's surgery, but then I decided I didn't want to take any risks. The duty doctor was based at a local hospital, and he explained he couldn't visit us for a while, but that if I took Lily there he could see her right away. Fortunately I have a car, so off we went. When we got to the doctor, Lily had perked up somewhat, perhaps because of being moved, so she was able to sit up and even smiled at the doctor. I was pleased as I thought she was getting better. The doctor looked at the spots, which he thought could be early chicken pox. He told me to take her home, give her paracetamol to reduce her temperature and call again if she got worse.

At first after seeing the doctor, Lily picked up. She had a little snack and then we watched a children's film on TV. Later, however, she vomited again and seemed to be very sleepy. I thought the chicken pox was wiping her out and that she would benefit from a good night's rest. I noticed that her temperature had gone up, and thought I would take her to the doctor again the next day as I was quite inexperienced dealing with illness.

When I went to Lily the next morning she felt very hot, and when I tried to wake her, her eyes looked glazed over. I couldn't keep her awake, and began to feel very worried. Then I looked at her spots and noticed that while the majority had gone, three deep red spots were still there. This immediately worried me. Without a lot of spots I thought it couldn't be chicken pox, and by the sick condition of my daughter, I knew it was something more serious. The possibility of meningitis floated across my mind. I knew I had to take action, and I rang the doctor again. I was asked to bring Lily straight round to the surgery, where she would be seen straight away. As we got ready to go out I was feeling panicky, fighting off fears of losing Lily, but as I moved her to get her dressed she again became more like herself, though she didn't like being moved and moaned about going out, so that I swung over to hoping I wasn't wasting the doctor's time.

Lily woke up a little as the doctor started examining her, but he was very concerned about her high temperature, her very cold hands and feet, her general floppiness, and the red spots I pointed out. He said he wanted us to go to the hospital straight away as he was concerned she might have meningitis. He gave Lily a jab of Penicillin, called an ambulance for us, and rang the hospital to alert them that we were on the way.

Comment

Lily had septicaemia caused by meningococcal bacteria. Fortunately she made a complete recovery.

At the start of Lily's illness, both her mother and the doctor quite reasonably thought she was coming down with an infection like chicken pox. Tiredness, lack of interest in things and a rash are early signs of many common virus infections in children, nearly all of which get better on their own, and when she was first seen by the doctor she had perked up and did not seem seriously ill. Her mother, keeping a close eye on her, felt things had changed by the next morning. The worrying things were her much greater drowsiness, her "glazed over" state, her high temperature with cold hands and feet, and the change in the spots, with most of them now gone but just three deep red ones to be seen. Despite her worry that she might be "wasting the doctor's time" as Lily seemed better for a while, Lily's mother took her to the doctor urgently. Far from wasting anyone's time, her action may have saved Lily's life. The doctor was immediately worried about meningitis, gave an injection of penicillin antibiotic and got Lily to hospital in an ambulance.

Parents must follow their instincts if they think their children are seriously ill. No parents should ever feel that they are wasting time if they contact the doctor with worries like these.

The table adjacent is a reminder of the features of meningitis and septicaemia caused by meningococcal bacteria. The ticks mark Lily's symptoms and signs.

Lily, aged 3	
High temperature	✔
Vomiting	✔
Pains in muscles and joints	
Weakness	✔
Severe headache	
Stiff neck	
Dislikes bright lights	
Drowsy or Confused	✔
Fits	
Cold/pale/blotchy skin	
Red/purple spots or bruises	✔

Introduction to Henry's and Ashley's stories.

The last two stories, Henry's and Ashley's, are very sad. Both little boys died of very rapid and severe septicaemia caused by meningococcal bacteria, and it is hard to see what could possibly have been done to save them. Their mothers have asked us to pass on their stories to make the point as strongly as possible what a terrible infection meningococcal bacteria can cause. They hope that their experience might help other parents to get over any hesitation to trouble the doctor for advice if they are worried about their children, and that other children's lives might thus be saved.

Henry, aged 2 years 8 months. His mother's story

At 4 o'clock in the afternoon I took Hen to the chemist to buy a bottle of paracetamol as he seemed heavy with a cold. He got out of the buggy and chose a packet of sweets.

We went through the park on the way home and fed the squirrels.

At 5 o'clock we went to Mum's and had something to eat. At 6 o'clock he dozed off to sleep, but at 7.30 he woke up and asked for a drink of water. He brought it right back up. We decided he didn't look well so we called the doctor. While we were waiting I lifted his sweatshirt to take his temperature and noticed three little spots at his waist. The thought of meningitis crossed my mind but I dismissed it thinking that it only happens to other people: after all, children get all kinds of rashes. Then Mum said his lips looked blue and he didn't look at all well. I phoned the doctor again and said that we were going to take Hen straight to the hospital.

We arrived at about 8 o'clock and were taken straight to the treatment room where Hen was given penicillin. By now he was obviously really ill and the team of doctors and nurses were doing all they could to stop the disease rampaging through his body, but there was nothing they could do.

Comment

Despite all that could be done, Hen became sicker and sicker, and died two hours later.

Ashley, aged 2 years 11 months. His mother's story

My husband Ian and I were on a three-day weekend break with my parents, my sister, and our two children, Ashley and Steven. On Saturday we all had a really busy day. We took the boys on a speed boat, played on the beach, spent the afternoon at a funfair, and in the evening we went to the holiday club at the camp site. The boys went to bed in the caravan at about 10.30.

Around four in the morning, Ashley woke up saying that his left leg was hurting him. He had rosy cheeks and felt a bit hot, which I put down to a touch of sunstroke. I gave him some paracetamol and had him in bed with us for about an hour and then lifted him into his own bed at around 5am, asleep.

When we all woke up at about quarter to nine, I checked on Ashley who was just stirring. He still had a slight temperature and complained that his leg hurt. I asked my mum and my sister to come and have a look, and between us we thought it best to take him to the local hospital to see why his leg was hurting. I thought he might have twisted it or trodden on something on the beach the day before, although there was no sign of swelling. I gave

Ashley another dose of paracetamol before dressing him and taking him to the local cottage hospital. Ashley was slightly sick after the paracetamol, although he didn't seem at all seriously ill.

We arrived at the hospital a while before the doctor came on duty, around eleven o'clock. The nurse found Ashley had quite a high temperature, and told us to take his dungarees off and cool him off with a damp cloth whilst we waited for the doctor. I told them Ashley had vomited his paracetamol back so they gave him another dose.

Ashley was talking to us about various Disney posters that were stuck up around the hospital walls. He said he was thirsty so my husband walked to the local store and brought him a can of Tango pop. I was also thirsty and had a sip but Ashley told me off for drinking his pop. He was perfectly coherent and alert.

The doctor checked Ashley over thoroughly, couldn't find anything wrong with his leg, but diagnosed tonsillitis and prescribed some antibiotics. He let us go home, but asked us to phone back later that afternoon to report on Ashley's condition, or if we were worried, to bring Ashley back to the hospital. I was glad to leave as I wanted to get Ashley back to the caravan and nurse him myself. He was getting sleepier and sleepier, though he was still answering when we talked to him. After a restless night and being prodded about in the hospital, I thought I would run him a cool bath, give him plenty of cuddles and lay him down for a rest.

I laid Ashley on the caravan seat, and set about running him a small bath. Ian and I were idly chatting about what to have for lunch and appreciating that Mum had left us the Sunday papers. I took Ashley's tee-shirt and underpants off and put him into the bath.

Nothing, nothing in the world, could have prepared us for the roller coaster ride we were about to embark on. As I lowered Ashley into the bath I saw about five bruise marks on his shoulder. They were the same bluey colour as the large veins are in my forearms. I looked at my listless, ill boy and suddenly I just knew what was wrong. "He's got meningitis" I screamed to Ian. High temperature, muscle pains, drowsiness, vomiting... but hold on, what about the "big indicators"; what about the stiff neck and dislike of bright lights. Ashley certainly didn't have these two symptoms - could I be over-reacting? Then I remembered how Mum had always said that the quieter a sick child is, the more worrying it is. I grabbed Ashley up, wrapped him in the bath towel and fled to the car. We screeched away leaving everything as it was. In my panic I'd got Ashley on my lap in the front seat of the car. I virtually had his head out of the window trying to keep him awake. I frantically chatted to him about the funfair ... anything to keep his eyes open and keep him talking to me.

As soon as we arrived, I ran with Ashley through the small hospital doors: my screaming brought immediate attention from the nurses. I was begging for them to phone for an ambulance and to fetch the doctor back who had originally seen Ashley. The room was spinning as I was fighting for breath in my panic. Ian took Ashley from me and showed him those wretched Disney posters again. Ashley just wanted to go to sleep, but Ian kept pressing him to answer his questions - "Is this poster the Lion King, Ashley?" - desperate to keep him alert.

The doctor arrived ten minutes later and gave Ashley a dose of intravenous Penicillin. Very soon the ambulance arrived, and Ashley was carried off still wrapped in his bath towel. I was allowed to travel with him on that awful fifteen minute journey. I knew he was desperately ill and I'd already convinced myself he would die. But then I'd think I was just being silly; there was Ashley still talking to me. He said he was hungry and wanted a biscuit. I breathed a sigh of relief - he had an appetite! But still, during that manic drive to the hospital I knew in my heart that Ashley was deteriorating. I could see his colour changing by the second. By now he had a purple-red rash, and if I looked away just for a moment, to blank out what was happening, when I looked back the rash would have spread even more. Imagine pouring beetroot juice onto the table cloth, then watching it spread and spoil the tablecloth. That was how it was with my little Ashley, he was spoiling by the second.

Comment.

Despite every effort at the hospital to save him, Ashley died later that afternoon.

CHAPTER 3

Part 1 of this chapter - What are meningitis and septicaemia? - explains in detail what these conditions are and how they occur. In part 2 - What germs cause meningitis? - the different viruses and bacteria that can cause the disease are described in detail, while in part 3 - Who gets meningitis, and why? - the relationship of meningitis risk to age, to the time of year and to other possible contributory factors is described.

Part 1:

What are meningitis and septicaemia?

What are meningitis and septicaemia? - key points

- Meningitis is inflammation of the membranes that cover the brain.

- Most serious cases of meningitis are caused by bacteria. Viruses generally cause much milder infections.

- The bacteria usually responsible for meningitis often exist harmlessly in the nose and throat but occasionally spread into the bloodstream and from there to the brain.

- In septicaemia, bacteria multiply in the blood causing widespread damage throughout the body. Septicaemia is a common and particularly serious problem in infections caused by meningococcal bacteria.

MENINGITIS

Meningitis means inflammation of the membranes - called the meninges - which cover the brain and spinal cord. The disease is usually caused by an infection with one of the two main types of germs that cause human diseases: viruses or bacteria. These are described in detail in part 2 *(page 60)*. Meningitis caused by viruses is generally thought to be commoner than that caused by bacteria, though this is based on a general impression rather than firm data as many cases of the viral form are never reported. It is usually quite a mild illness and many cases are probably never recognised as meningitis at all, instead being diagnosed, for example, as a nasty dose of flu with sickness and a bad headache. Though it can be very unpleasant at the time, meningitis caused by viruses usually resolves on its own without leaving any long term damage. This is very fortunate as with few exceptions there are no drugs to treat these infections: antibiotics are only effective against bacteria. It is fortunate too that meningitis caused by bacteria is rarer, as it is a much more serious illness. Without adequate treatment with powerful antibiotics and, in the most serious cases, life support in an intensive care unit, it can cause permanent brain damage or death.

Figure 1. The brain, spinal cord and meninges - see facing page

The spinal cord extends down the back from the brain, within the spinal canal which is filled with cerebrospinal fluid. Nerve fibres pass out from the spinal cord to the tissues through the meninges.

A. Enlargement showing (i) brain; (ii) space where the cerebrospinal fluid flows; (iii) outer layer of meninges; (iv) bone of the skull, with the scalp above it.

B. Enlargement showing how the space containing cerebrospinal fluid continues from around the base of the brain to around the spinal cord.

C. Enlargement showing the lower end of the spinal cord. There is space containing cerebrospinal fluid and nerve fibres below the spinal cord, where a needle (marked with arrowhead) may safely be inserted for a lumbar puncture test (see *page 76*).

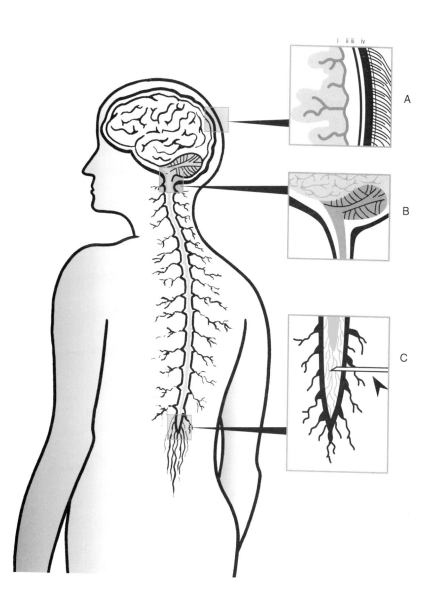

Within the skull, the meninges form a tough covering for the brain which extends down the spine to cover the spinal cord as well. (see figure 1). Together with the skull and spine, the meninges protect the brain and spinal cord from physical damage. Under the meninges there is a colourless, watery liquid called cerebrospinal fluid. Cerebrospinal fluid is produced in reservoirs inside the brain *(see figure 4, page 78)*. It passes freely out from these reservoirs through gaps at the base of the brain to flow over its surface beneath the meninges, from where it is later taken up into the bloodstream. Cerebrospinal fluid circulates both over the brain surface and down the spine, providing a shock-absorbing cushion around the whole brain and spinal cord (see figure 1).

Cerebrospinal fluid is normally completely protected from infection. The tough meninges make a barrier that stops bacteria entering from the outside world. Bacteria are prevented from spreading in through the bloodstream by the action of the body's immune system which detects, attacks and destroys them. If, however, bacteria ever *do* succeed in overcoming these defences and get into the cerebrospinal fluid, there is nothing there to stop them multiplying rapidly, and the infected fluid can spread all over the brain and spinal cord. ***This is the basic problem in meningitis.***

How bacteria get to the meninges and through them to cause meningitis.

Three varieties of bacteria - the "big three" - are found again and again causing cases of meningitis: meningococcal bacteria, pneumococcal bacteria and Hib bacteria. One or other of these three varieties can very often be found in the secretions of the nose or throat of people who are entirely well. Occasionally the bacteria may cause minor infections like sore throat, sinusitis or earache. However, very rarely, they can break through the lining of the nose, the throat, or the middle ear, and get into the bloodstream. Once there,there is a small risk that they will overwhelm the body's defences and build up to high numbers in the blood. The bacteria may then spread through the body to the brain. In the brain they may damage the delicate blood vessels of the meninges to create microscopic openings through which they can get into the cerebrospinal fluid and cause meningitis.

In rare cases, the route by which bacteria get to the cerebrospinal fluid is much more direct. For example, meningitis can result from bacteria getting in with dirt into a skull fracture after an accident, or it may very occasionally occur if bacteria get in at the time of brain or spinal surgery. Rarely, a baby may be born with a defect in the way the bones and covering skin of the skull or spine have grown together so that a tiny gap remains. In these circumstances, germs from the skin, from behind the ear drums or from the sinuses can penetrate to the cerebrospinal fluid and cause meningitis.

What happens once germs reach the cerebrospinal fluid.

If germs do manage to enter the cerebrospinal fluid, there is little to stop them multiplying at a very great rate: the bacteria may double their numbers every half hour. As they do so, they release poisonous substances which damage the delicate tissues and tiny blood vessels on the brain surface. A chain reaction of events termed inflammation is triggered, in which further poisons released by the body's own injured cells lead to more and more damage. The same process is familiar in everyday life when a cut becomes infected. The warmth and redness that are seen reflect the dilating of blood vessels as they bring cells that fight infection to the site. Swelling occurs as the damaged cells and tissues leak fluid into the surrounding area; and pain follows as poisons in the infected region irritate sensitive nerve endings. In meningitis all these events are taking place on a large scale, not just at the point that the infection gets in, but all over the surface of the brain.

How inflammation causes the symptoms and signs of meningitis.

The inflammation caused by the infection irritates nerve endings in the meninges and causes a severe headache. The muscles of the neck tighten in spasm and the neck becomes stiff, and very painful to bend. Headache also occurs as a result of swelling of the meninges and the brain beneath. This swelling is resisted by the bones of the skull, and as a result the brain is put under pressure. In babies where the bones of the skull have not yet grown together completely, the soft spot towards the front of the top of the head - the fontanelle - may bulge out as a result of the pressure. However, increased pressure on the brain and the nerve cell damage caused by the inflammation can have far more serious consequences than just causing a severe headache. Inflammation and pressure at the base of the brain leads to a feeling of sickness and may cause vomiting. It affects the way the nerves to the internal muscles of the eye work, causing pain on exposure to bright lights. Most important of all, it can affect the fundamental workings of the brain, and lead to confusion and drowsiness, or a fit *(see box, page 15)*. If the disease progresses further, increasing brain swelling can lead to dangerously high pressure within the skull, which causes increasing drowsiness and eventually loss of consciousness (coma). The functioning of vital parts of the brain involved in breathing and the blood circulation becomes threatened, and only emergency treatment can prevent death.

SEPTICAEMIA

In septicaemia (also known as blood poisoning), bacteria infect the blood, spreading through the bloodstream to make the patient ill. In healthy people of all ages, the body's defences against infection are very efficient at ensuring that bacteria do not multiply in the blood to the point that they cause problems. Septicaemia is therefore very rare except in those with weakened defences against infection: the very elderly, for example, or some cancer patients, or people with AIDS. Septicaemia may however occur in healthy people when bacteria are involved which are particularly hard for the body's immune system to detect or to kill. This applies to all of the "big three" meningitis bacteria. Of these, meningococcal bacteria are the commonest to cause dangerous septicaemia, a widespread infection in which many organs of the body may be damaged. For reasons which are not understood, the extent to which meningococcal bacteria produce this damage is very variable. At worst, the septicaemia causes very severe illness, which may rapidly lead to death (as in Henry's and Ashley's cases described in chapter 2), while other cases may be much milder (like Noora's case *page 41)*. The meningococcal bacteria multiply in the bloodstream and release poisons which cause inflammation all over the body, making small blood vessels everywhere leaky. Fluid seeps out of the damaged blood vessels so that there is less blood available for the heart to pump around the body, causing the heart rate to increase and the blood pressure to fall. Some of the poisons impair the normal functioning of the heart so that it pumps less effectively and the blood pressure falls still more. As these problems build up, the skin, muscle, internal organs and brain become starved of blood and oxygen. As blood is diverted away from the skin, the victim becomes very pale and cold. Blood may leak out of damaged blood vessels in the surface layers of the skin, leading to dark red spots or marks like love-bites or bruises appearing. These may get very large if advancing infection stops the blood clotting properly. As the muscles become starved of blood, painful aches and cramps may develop. The reduction in the blood supply to the brain results in confusion and later drowsiness and eventually unconsciousness. Later blood may be diverted away from internal organs to the extent that they stop working properly. While all these problems are building up, the bacteria can spread from the bloodstream to many parts of the body, including the brain. Meningitis commonly occurs alongside meningococcal septicaemia: six out of ten victims will have both conditions.

Part 2:
What germs cause meningitis?

What germs cause meningitis? - Key Points

- Most cases of meningitis are caused by two kinds of germ: viruses and bacteria.

- Viral meningitis is commoner, and a less severe illness than bacterial meningitis. Viral meningitis nearly always resolves completely without special treatment.

- Bacterial meningitis is rarer and much more severe than viral meningitis. A small number of varieties of bacteria are responsible for most cases, and these are the same germs that usually live harmlessly in the nose or throat. The commonest germ causing bacterial meningitis and septicaemia in the UK is the meningococcus.

Most cases of meningitis are caused by two kinds of germ: viruses and bacteria. Both these germs are much smaller than the cells that make up our bodies. If a person were enlarged to the size of the UK, his individual cells would be about the size of a car, bacteria on his skin would only be the size of a paving stone, while a typical virus might be the size of a fifty pence coin lying in the gutter.

Infections caused by viruses

Viruses are tiny infectious particles, so rudimentary in nature that they cannot multiply outside the cells of living things. There are many kinds of viruses, responsible for most of the common illnesses which afflict us. The common cold, flu, many sore throats and ear infections, many cases of vomiting and diarrhoea, measles, mumps, german measles (rubella), chicken pox ... these are all virus infections.

Some of the viruses which cause colds, diarrhoea and so forth are also capable of spreading through the body to the brain and meninges, to cause viral meningitis. The signs and symptoms are the same as those of meningitis caused by bacteria, but the disease is usually much less severe, and serious complications are very unusual.

In most cases where a virus is thought to be responsible for a case of meningitis, the exact variety is never discovered. In the cases where a virus *is* identified, it is usually one of the enterovirus family. Enterovirus infections most frequently occur in the summer and autumn months, mainly taking the form of diarrhoea, sore throats, coughs and colds, but occasionally meningitis. Enteroviruses are passed around from an infected person in droplets during sneezing and coughing and on unwashed hands. Spread between young children and within families is common. The incubation period (between picking up the virus and developing the illness) is between four and six days. Infections caused by enteroviruses (including meningitis) generally get completely better without complications. The exception, in those places where it still causes problems, is polio virus. This is different from the other enteroviruses in sometimes causing a far more severe disease (poliomyelitis) in which permanent nerve damage and paralysis may occur. Polio vaccine, given to all children in the UK at 2, 3 and 4 months of age, again before school, and periodically after that, is extremely effective in preventing polio and there is a hope that with its use all over the world, polio will be extinct by the year 2000.

Until recently, the next most common virus identified as the cause of meningitis in the UK was mumps virus. Like meningitis caused by enteroviruses, mumps virus meningitis is usually a brief though unpleasant illness which gets better, leaving no after effects, though occasionally a more severe infection of the brain may occur with the complication of deafness. The measles, mumps and rubella vaccine (MMR), given to children in the UK at 12-15 months, is effective in preventing mumps infections including meningitis (see chapter 8).

A variety of herpes virus (known as herpes simplex virus type 2) causes a sexually-transmitted infection known as genital herpes, but it can also cause meningitis. As many as three in ten people having a first attack of genital herpes may have meningitis at the same time. Treatment with the drug aciclovir is possible in cases of herpes simplex virus infections. Aciclovir is one of the few medications available which can kill viruses, and in meningitis this is usually given in hospital as a course of injections into the bloodstream through an intravenous drip.

Table 3. Viruses which cause meningitis in the U.K.

Virus	More usual illness than meningitis	Possibilities for prevention and treatment
Enteroviruses	Colds, Sore throats, Diarrhoea	Care with hygiene, especially hand washing. Polio vaccine protects against polio virus infections, but not other enteroviruses.
Mumps virus	Mumps	MMR vaccine protects
Herpes simplex virus type 2	Genital herpes	Treatment possible with the antiviral drug aciclovir.

Infections caused by bacteria

Bacteria exist everywhere around us in the environment. Most varieties are harmless. Our skin, our mouths, noses and throats, and the lower part of the digestive tract, are teeming with bacteria with which we live, for the most part, in complete harmony. These bacteria pass regularly from one person to another in the course of everyday life, in coughs and sneezes and on our hands, so that as the years pass we meet a great many different sorts. Our body's immune system is strengthened by this constant exposure, and the result is that as we grow from childhood into adult life, we become less prone to infections.

Of the tiny minority of bacteria that causes any problems at all in humans, only a small proportion regularly causes serious infection. Most of the bacteria that do cause problems generally do little long term harm because they do not spread deep into the body. In a typical infection like a boil, a sore throat or an earache, the germs remain localised in one place until the body's defence mechanisms destroy them. However, on very rare occasions, a localised infection (which may be very minor indeed) may progress to a much more serious illness in which bacteria overwhelm the body's defences and spread widely. Much research is directed at trying to understand why in rare instances bacteria behave in this way. While it is not completely understood, one important factor has been identified. All the "big three" meningitis bacteria, and most others that can cause meningitis, have a special slimy outer coat which protects them from being readily detected and killed by the body's defences. If they reach the bloodstream, this coat makes it more likely that these bacteria will multiply there in an unrestricted fashion. In some cases it has been possible to develop vaccines based on this coat which can prevent meningitis (see chapter 8).

Table 4. The main varieties of bacteria that cause meningitis

In babies over 1 month of age, children and adults:
The "big three":   Meningococcal bacteria
Pneumococcal bacteria
Hib bacteria

In newborn infants:
Group B streptococcal bacteria
Coliform bacteria
Listeria bacteria

Meningococcal bacteria

Meningococcal bacteria are now the commonest cause of bacterial meningitis in the UK. About 1500 cases of meningococcal disease are reported by doctors in England and Wales each year, though the true total that occurs is almost certainly higher than this as some cases inevitably fail to reach the official figures. However, to put that number in perspective, at any one time one in ten people have these bacteria living harmlessly in the nose or throat - that is, more than five million people in the UK are carrying the germ at this very moment. Nearly everyone becomes immune as a result of carrying germs in this way *(see page 68)* virtually eliminating their risk of meningitis as they get older. The likelihood that people will be carrying meningococcal bacteria in the nose and throat changes with age. Children under five years old are not often carriers, but teenagers are carriers very commonly: one in four carry them. Almost everyone who carries the germ is unaware of the fact, and never gets ill. On the rare occasions that meningococcal bacteria do cause problems, however, the infection begins three to ten days after the germ is passed to the victim. In the UK most of these cases happen in the winter months, when germs can spread widely through close contact between people. This can occur in droplets produced in coughs and sneezes, probably on fingers that have rubbed noses, and directly by kissing on the lips.

There are three main sorts of meningococcal bacteria, termed serogroup A, serogroup B and serogroup C strains. Each of these has a different sort of slimy outer coat which makes it difficult for the immune system to detect and kill it. The serogroup B coat is particularly difficult for the human immune system to deal with, and cases of disease caused by serogroup B strains are the commonest in the UK, causing seven out of ten meningococcal bacterial infections. Serogroup C strains cause the rest. Serogroup A strains only very rarely cause problems in the UK, but are a major cause of illness in some developing countries (see chapter 7). These three strains do not differ in the diseases they produce (meningococcal meningitis and septicaemia).

Pneumococcal bacteria

Pneumococcal bacteria are among the commonest to cause chest infections and ear infections, but they can also cause meningitis. There are about 200 cases of meningitis caused by pneumococcal bacteria reported in England and Wales each year, mostly occurring in the winter. Like the other bacteria that cause meningitis, pneumococcal bacteria are also carried in the nose and throat, and they are spread in a similar way to the rest. There are nearly a hundred different types of pneumococcal bacteria, distinguished by their slimy outer coat, which can cause meningitis, but in the UK seven types are responsible for most of the infections.

Hib bacteria

Until 1992, meningitis caused by Hib bacteria was almost as common in the UK as meningococcal disease. There were about 1300 cases reported each year by doctors in England and Wales. Like meningococcal bacteria, Hib is commonly found in the noses and throats of healthy individuals. Children under five years old are the most likely to be carrying the germ. Probably almost all of them have done so by that age. Like meningococcal bacteria, each Hib germ has a slimy coating on the surface which helps it survive in the bloodstream. From there the Hib bacteria can spread to the brain to cause meningitis. Since 1992 the picture in the UK has changed dramatically. A very effective vaccine, the Hib vaccine, has been given routinely to all children (see chapter 8), and prevented most cases of Hib meningitis. There were less than fifty cases reported in England and Wales in the year to mid-1996.

Bacteria causing meningitis in newborn infants

If newborn babies get meningitis, the germs involved are usually different from those affecting older children (see table 4, page 63). Newborn babies are mainly at risk of infection from bacteria that they acquire from their mothers at the time of birth. These are the bacteria that generally exist harmlessly in everyone's digestive tract and genital region. Two varieties are particularly associated with meningitis: coliform bacteria from the bowel, and group B streptococcal bacteria from the genital region.

Infection of the baby may occur before birth or during delivery. In some cases when the waters break a long time before the baby is born, the fluid surrounding the baby may become infected. The bacteria can spread to the baby so that it is born with meningitis or other severe infection. In other cases infection begins during delivery. As the baby passes out of the birth canal and gives the first gasps, bacteria get into the mouth and throat. Usually no harm comes of this, but on rare occasions they may break through into the bloodstream. Once again these bacteria have slimy outer coats which increase the chance that they will survive long enough to reach the brain and meninges and cause meningitis. There are about one hundred cases of meningitis and septicaemia caused by these bacteria reported in newborn babies in England and Wales each year.

Listeria is another variety of bacterial germ which can exist in the human digestive tract and which may rarely cause meningitis in newborn babies. The infection that Listeria causes in a pregnant woman is usually mild, with little more than a fever, but the bacteria can spread to the baby before birth to affect it much more severely. Listeria can be found in unpasteurised dairy products such as soft cheeses, and in processed meats like paté. Although the chance of mother or baby getting a Listeria infection is very small, women are now advised to avoid these foods during pregnancy to minimise the risk.

Part 3:
Who gets meningitis, and why?

Who gets meningitis, and why? - Key Points

- Meningitis caused by bacteria is commonest from six months to two years of age, and the risk falls rapidly as children get older.

- There is a small increase in risk again for infection caused by meningococcal bacteria in young adult years, and in old age for infections with pneumococcal bacteria.

- More cases of bacterial meningitis and meningococcal septicaemia occur in the winter than at other times of the year.

- Some rare genetic abnormalities, diseases that depress the immune system, recent flu virus infection and smoking have all been shown to increase the risk of bacterial meningitis to some extent.

Age

Although meningitis caused by viruses or bacteria can strike at any age, it is mainly a disease of children and young people. For infections caused by each of the "big three" meningitis bacteria (table 4) described on pages 63-65, the risk is comparatively small at birth, greatest in babies over six months, and gets less with increasing age. This variation in risk with age is shown in figure 2, for cases of disease caused by meningococcal bacteria.

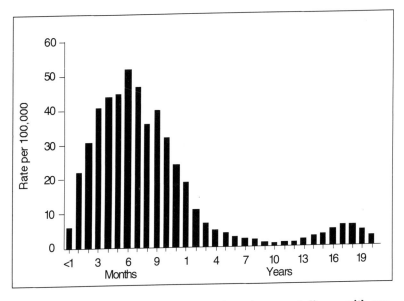

Figure 2. Variation in number of cases of meningococcal disease with age. Figures for England and Wales, 1984 - 1991. Bars show the average number of cases per 100,000 children of each of the ages shown per year.

The reason for this variation in risk with age lies in the way that the body's immune system works to fight infection. Antibodies in the blood are a very important part of the immune system protecting against meningitis bacteria. Antibodies are made every time we come into contact with the meningitis germs themselves or others closely related to them. As described on page 56, meningitis bacteria commonly live in the nose and throat where they generally cause no harm at all. All the same, the body's immune system detects them there, and antibodies are made which then protect against the possibility that the germs might invade. Protection also builds up as a result of the similarity between meningitis bacteria and other harmless bacteria which naturally exist in our bodies, for example in the digestive tract. The body's immune system responds to these as if they might be meningitis germs, and defences against meningitis are boosted as a result.

Before birth, antibodies are passed from a mother to her baby in the womb.

At birth a baby is therefore quite well protected against the "big three" meningitis bacteria, so that they only rarely cause infections in the first months of life. During the first six months, however, the mother's antibodies in the baby's blood dwindle away, so that between six and eight months of age the risk of infections caused by meningitis bacteria is at its highest. At that time the mother's antibodies have disappeared from the baby's blood, and the baby has developed little resistance of his/her own. All the while, however, the baby is manufacturing antibodies as more and more varieties of germs are encountered, so that from this low point things improve. However, the ability to make protective antibodies against the "big three" meningitis bacteria does not develop fully until about two years of age and, until then, young children remain at greater risk than older children and adults. This increase in resistance to infection with age is reflected in a falling rate of disease, as was shown for meningococcal infection (meningitis and septicaemia) in figure 2 *(page 68)*.

Even before the Hib vaccine for children was introduced (see chapter 8), by the time a child reached the age of 5 years, the risk of getting Hib meningitis had virtually disappeared. By that age almost all children had become well protected by their own antibodies, made as a result of natural exposure to Hib bacteria or similar harmless germs. For meningitis and septicaemia caused by meningococcal bacteria, the risk after the first few years of life is less than in the first year or two, but it does not reduce as rapidly, or to quite as low a level, as is seen with Hib meningitis. Indeed, there is a slight increase in risk again in the teenage years *(figure 2, page 68)*. This is at least partly explained by the wider range of meningococcal bacteria compared to the single variety of Hib germ that causes meningitis (see chapter 8), so that it takes longer to make antibodies to protect against all varieties. Another reason why the rate of meningococcal bacterial infections increases a little in teenagers may be the lifestyle changes that are a part of growing up. Close contact between teenagers in schools, clubs, camps and college halls of residence leads to germs spreading widely between people outside the family, so that teenagers are meeting a whole range of new strains for the first time.

The risk of meningitis caused by pneumococcal bacteria, like the rest, is clearly related to age, with a peak in babies, falling to a very low risk through adult life. There is however a rise again in risk in the elderly, with the disease becoming slightly more common again in over-seventy-year -olds.

In response to widespread concerns about the risk of meningitis, a great deal of research effort has gone into trying to identify factors that increase the chance that someone might develop the disease. Researchers have examined factors in the patients themselves, and factors in people's lifestyles and in their environment.

Inherited and acquired factors

As the immune system is so important in protecting against meningitis, it is not surprising that conditions in which it is not functioning properly are associated with an increased risk. New examples of such conditions are continually being discovered, though each of them is very rare indeed. Some are inherited and others acquired during life.

In one rare inherited condition there is an increased risk particularly of infection with meningococcal bacteria. In this condition there is a deficiency of one of a family of proteins in the blood known as Complement, which assist antibodies in killing germs, especially meningococcal bacteria. About 1 in 3000 people have a deficiency of Complement, and they are more prone to meningococcal disease than the population in general. Half of them are likely to have meningococcal infection at some time in their lives, and they may have more than one attack. Many paediatricians will arrange a blood test to check the Complement proteins in patients who have had meningococcal disease - certainly in anyone who has had it more than once - as those who are discovered to have defects can be alerted to their susceptibility and protected with antibiotics.

Among acquired conditions which increase the risk of meningitis - all of which are also rare - one of the most frequent is a progressive failure of the spleen to work properly. The spleen is an internal organ, forming part of the immune system, that is particularly important in protecting against infection of the blood by meningitis bacteria. Children with various rare inherited blood conditions, including sickle cell anaemia, for example, commonly have spleens which cease to work effectively by the end of their first year, and they are then prone to infection with pneumococcal bacteria in particular. The spleen may also be damaged and have to be removed after an accident, or in the treatment of some kinds of cancer. Whatever the reason, the antibiotic medicine penicillin is often prescribed in a daily dose to children without a spleen to protect them against severe infections including meningitis, and vaccinations are offered for added protection (see chapter 8). Diseases such as cancer, leukaemia or lymphoma, and the treatments used for them, make sufferers prone to bacterial infections of all kinds, including meningitis. AIDS sufferers too are at increased risk of septicaemia and bacterial meningitis.

The special risk for meningitis associated with an abnormal gap in the meninges, allowing germs to get in from the sinuses, the back of the throat or behind the ear drum, has already been mentioned *(page 57)*.

Lifestyle and environment

There have been many scares about risks associated with different lifestyles or environmental factors, but on closer scrutiny most have never been *proved* to increase the risk of meningitis. The difficulty is that there are nearly always several plausible explanations for the observations that have been made, and it can be impossible to say which, if any, of them are correct. Despite this, research is often misrepresented to suggest that a particular factor is linked to meningitis, even though the findings are far from conclusive.

A recent example occurred in September 1996, when scientists reported that there had been more cases of disease caused by meningococcal bacteria in an area where doctors prescribed more of one common antibiotic than in areas where less was prescribed. There was an immediate response in the media, raising the alarm that dangerous "superbugs", resistant to antibiotics, might have been created by too much antibiotic prescribing by GPs.

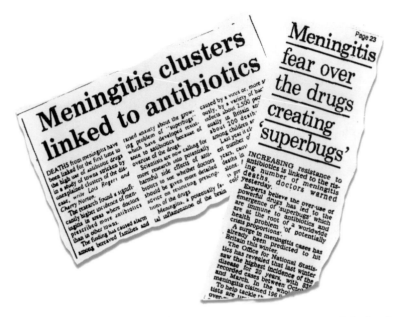

What the researchers actually reported was that when they reviewed the local records of cases of meningitis from nearly ten years before, they found that there had been more prescribing of the antibiotic in question in a district with more cases than in an area otherwise similar where the rate of infection was low. There has been *no* increase in resistance of the germs to that antibiotic, which in any case is not used to treat infections caused by meningococcal bacteria, ruling out the "superbug" idea. The significance of their interesting observation is still unexplained.

Among things that have been shown in careful studies to be associated with an increased rate of meningitis are:

Minor virus infections

It is often noticed that cases of meningitis caused by bacteria are preceded by coughs, colds, and ear ache. This has led to the question of whether infection with the viruses that cause such illnesses might increase the risk of meningitis, in some way weakening the system and letting bacteria get in. A weak link has been found between infection with meningococcal bacteria and flu virus infections, but no link to other cough and cold viruses.

The season of the year and the climate

Meningitis caused by viruses is more common in the Summer and Autumn months than at other times of year. This probably reflects the greater rate then of illnesses with the enteroviruses that are an important cause of viral meningitis *(see pages 60-62)*. In contrast, in both the Northern and Southern hemispheres, meningitis caused by bacteria is much commoner in the cold wet winter months. The association may possibly be explained by the increased rate of colds and flu, and the increased likelihood that people will mix indoors and spread infection in coughs and sneezes. Near the equator, in the African Meningitis Belt (see chapter 7), there is a great increase in the number of cases of meningitis caused by meningococcal bacteria during the dry season. It has been suggested that this is because the linings of the nose and throat get dry and inflamed at this time of year, allowing meningococcal germs to get through into the bloodstream. It has been wondered whether changes in atmospheric pressure might affect the risk of infection, but no good evidence has been found for this.

Smoking

Yet another reason for giving up smoking is that there is an association between it and meningitis. Children in households where parents smoke appear to be at a slightly increased risk of getting disease caused by meningococcal bacteria. Smoking also seems slightly to increase the risk of the smoker getting meningitis. The link may be through the damage that irritant cigarette smoke causes to the linings of the nose and throat, allowing meningitis germs to get in more easily.

Diet

The specific risk of meningitis in newborn infants caused by their mothers eating unpasteurised foods (dairy products, paté) contaminated with Listeria bacteria has been mentioned already *(see page 66)*. No other eating habits and no sorts of vitamin deficiency have been associated with meningitis, and there is no evidence that particular diets or diet supplementation can protect against infection.

In the end, it is important to keep things in a sensible perspective. Although they have a very high profile in the media, bacterial meningitis and meningococcal septicaemia are rare diseases. For example, the figures from 1993 show that you were more than five times more likely to have been killed in a car accident than your child was to die of bacterial meningitis or septicaemia.

CHAPTER 4
How is Meningitis Treated?

Introduction

If your child is unwell and you are worried you should contact your GP to ask for advice, saying that you are concerned about the possibility of meningitis. You may be reassured after talking to the doctor, who may visit, or ask you to bring your child to the surgery or health centre, or even to go straight to hospital. If on seeing your child the doctor thinks it possible that the diagnosis might be bacterial meningitis, or septicaemia caused by meningococcal bacteria, then he or she will often give an injection of antibiotic medicine immediately, and arrange for your child to be taken urgently to hospital.

The Accident and Emergency Department

On arrival at the Accident and Emergency Department (Casualty Department) the patient will quickly be seen by a nurse (the triage nurse) who decides how urgently a doctor is needed. In cases where meningitis is suspected or a child has been referred by the GP, the triage nurse may pass the patient on immediately to an accident and emergency doctor, or arrange for a specialist (for example a paediatrician) to come right away. Seriously ill patients may be seen by a team of doctors and nurses who make an assessment together and start treatment immediately. It all may appear very frightening but someone will come and explain what is going on in more detail as soon as all urgent treatment has been started.

The doctor will usually begin by making a quick assessment both to begin to sort out what is wrong and to decide if the patient might already be dangerously ill and in need of treatment without any further delay. The doctor will want to know all about symptoms, and how long the patient has been ill; about any other medical problems; and about the health of other members of the family and household contacts. The doctor will examine the patient looking for signs of meningitis and other serious illness, and may then arrange some tests. A lumbar puncture is one of the main investigations that can help to discover if someone has meningitis. This test usually allows the diagnosis to be made within hours, and may give important information as to which germ is responsible *(see plate 10, page 24)*, so allowing the best treatment to be given without delay. The doctor caring for the patient will decide when, or if, a lumbar puncture is to be done. The test may be carried out almost immediately, in the Accident and Emergency Department, or later, in the hospital ward.

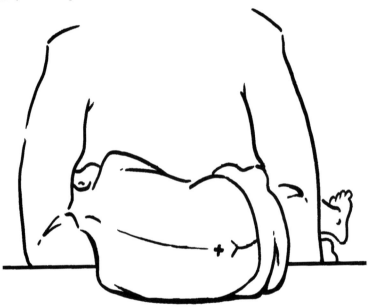

Figure 3. Baby being held for a lumbar puncture test.
The baby lying on a couch is held securely by a nurse so that he/she cannot move as the needle is inserted into the spinal canal (at the point marked with a cross) to collect a small sample of cerebrospinal fluid. (See also Figure 1).

For a lumbar puncture test to be carried out on a child, the patient is laid on one side, and held securely. A hollow needle is then inserted into the spinal canal in the lower back *(See Figure 1 (pages 54-55); Figure 3; plates 9 and 10 page 24))*. A little local anaesthetic may be used to numb the skin, and the test hurts no more than a blood test. Cerebrospinal fluid - the fluid that becomes infected in meningitis - drips out of the needle and is collected and taken straight to the hospital laboratory to be analysed. If the patient has not already had an injection of antibiotic medicine, this will usually be given shortly after the lumbar puncture.

Sometimes a lumbar puncture may not be done even when meningitis is suspected. This may be because the patient is seriously ill and in need of urgent treatment. In such cases the lumbar puncture can wait. Treatment with powerful antibiotics is started immediately, and the question of whether a lumbar puncture is needed is deferred until the patient's condition has improved.

The patient with meningitis on a hospital ward

While meningitis is always a serious illness, it is not usually life- threatening if treated promptly. Most patients with meningitis are admitted to a regular ward in the hospital for treatment, and parents are always encouraged to arrange for at least one parent to stay with their child. It may be that for the first 24 to 48 hours a child with meningitis will be nursed in a single room, isolated from other children ("barrier nursing"), but after having had antibiotic treatment for that time, there is no risk of passing infection on to others and the child can be nursed in any area of the ward. In cases of suspected meningitis or septicaemia caused by meningococcal bacteria, close family and household contacts will be given antibiotic medicine to reduce the risk of them becoming ill with the same infection (See chapter 6).

A child with bacterial meningitis will generally need to be looked after in hospital for at least one week, and often longer. The first couple of days and nights may be very busy and disturbed. The child is likely to be very drowsy or have many short naps, and may be miserable and irritable when awake. Through this period the nurses and doctors will be checking repeatedly that the child is not getting any worse - in particular, that the infection is coming under control and that there is no dangerous build up of pressure on the brain. To monitor this, the child's temperature, heart rate, breathing rate, blood pressure and level of consciousness will be recorded repeatedly - usually every four hours, but sometimes more frequently. In some cases the doctors may need to arrange a brain scan, or a recording of the patient's brain wave activity, especially if the child has had a fit.

To get a brain scan, the patient will need to be moved to the X-ray or Scanning Department of the hospital. Depending on exactly what is needed, the scan itself can take anything from a few minutes to half an hour. Although the procedure is painless, it is important for the patient to lie quite still while the scanning is being done, so a mild sedative, or sometimes even an anaesthetic, may be given. There are two different sorts of scans that might be taken. The more common is a CT scan (also sometimes called a CAT scan, short for Computerised Axial Tomography scan). This provides a detailed picture of the brain taken with X-rays, and shows up areas of inflammation, swelling, or possible complications of meningitis (*see plate 13, page 26, and Figure 4*). An MRI scan (standing for Magnetic Resonance Imaging scan) gives similar information but is obtained by the use of a high magnetic field rather than X-rays.

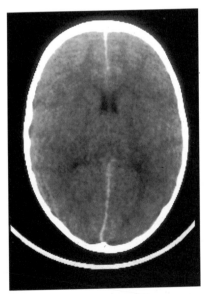

Figure 4. A CT scan.
A cross-sectional X-ray picture of the brain (in grey) and the central reservoirs (in black, in the middle of the brain) where cerebrospinal fluid is made.

A brain wave recording (an EEG, standing for electroencephalograph) can usually be done at the patient's bedside. Again this is a painless procedure, though it can be rather messy, as electrodes have to be fixed all over the patient's head with sticky gel *(plate 14, page 26)*. The electrical activity of the brain is picked up, amplified and traced on to a long roll of paper which is then taken away to be interpreted and reported by a specialist.

While these checks and investigations are being carried out, antibiotic medication will be being given as regular injections into an intravenous drip.

In many cases of meningitis caused by bacteria, patients begin to show clear signs of recovering by the third day or so. As the time in hospital continues, the early bustle can come to be replaced with much less attention from the doctors, as they spend more time with other, sicker, children. This is a good sign that things are getting better. The child may seem virtually back to normal, and it can be very hard to tolerate staying in hospital especially with a toddler who is missing home, hating the hospital room, and very hard to amuse. However, it may be necessary to keep on with the antibiotic treatment for a week or more after this improvement has taken place, as it is very important that every single germ is killed. If treatment is stopped too soon, the meningitis may return. For this reason, antibiotics are given for at least a week, and perhaps up to three weeks (depending on the particular variety of germ responsible for the meningitis). It may be possible for the doctors to switch the medication from an injectable form to syrup or capsules which can be taken by mouth. If that is not suitable, it might be possible to arrange for the last few days of treatment to be given by injections at home.

Severe cases of meningitis and septicaemia

Rarely, a case of meningitis gets so advanced that there are fears for the patient's life. Such patients may deteriorate quickly, having fits, losing consciousness, getting into difficulties breathing for themselves, or choking. Steps may quickly need to be taken to deal with these problems by starting intensive care. The patient may need to be connected to a ventilator machine to assist with breathing, and medication may have to be given to control fits and to reduce the swelling of the brain that may be causing these problems. A great deal will suddenly seem to be happening with many tubes attached to the patient, intravenous drips running into veins, and lots of wires connected to electronic monitors in order to keep a close check on vital organs such as the heart and lungs.

Patients with septicaemia caused by meningococcal bacteria can be very seriously ill, and may also very quickly need intensive care. Their immediate needs might include help with breathing from a ventilator machine, medications to stimulate the heart, medication to deal with fits, infusions of plasma into one or more intravenous drip to help keep up the blood pressure, as well as antibiotic medication to fight the infection. Serious problems can arise as the infection damages small blood vessels and larger veins. The skin and muscles can be very badly injured, so much so that emergency surgical treatment may be needed to save a limb. More complex treatments may be needed within a short space of time as vital organs are threatened by the infection. Such severely ill patients need treatment and monitoring with special equipment that is only available in an intensive care unit.

Transfer of critically ill children to an intensive care unit

If a child with suspected meningitis or septicaemia is very ill when brought to hospital, or appears to be getting worse in spite of treatment, the doctors may decide that specialised care is needed of the kind that can only be given in an intensive care unit. All major hospitals have intensive care units with facilities for adults where children can be cared for in an emergency. However specialised paediatric intensive care units - designed, equipped and staffed specifically for the care of very sick children - are not so widely available, and the doctors may decide that a child has to be transferred to the nearest such unit. If possible the transfer of a very sick child will be supervised by a mobile intensive care team of a specially trained doctor and nurse coming out by ambulance from the paediatric intensive care unit to collect the patient.

Before moving any child, the mobile intensive care team will do their best to help the local doctors make sure that the patient's condition is stable. The sicker a patient is when the mobile team arrives, the longer they are likely to spend working at the hospital before leaving. This initial period is very important as it is in this way that the chances of problems occurring in the ambulance during transfer are minimised. All the same, the ambulance is equipped for dealing with intensive care emergencies even while on the move. The team may spend several hours working with the local doctors to stabilise the patient. The sick child will then be connected to the mobile life support machine and monitors before embarking on the journey back to the paediatric intensive care unit by specialised ambulance or even, in some cases, by helicopter *(plates 11 and 12, page 25)*.

The paediatric intensive care unit

Severely ill patients are admitted to an intensive care unit so that their condition can be monitored very closely. Life support measures can be provided quickly, and treatment can be given to maintain the functioning of vital organs such as the heart, lungs, and kidneys.

An intensive care unit can seem a bewildering and frightening place, with equipment bleeping all the time, and each patient almost hidden beneath tubes and wires connected to machines. *(plate 15, page 27)*. Depending on a patient's particular condition, a large range of investigations, procedures, and even operations, can be carried out on the unit. If necessary, a patient can be moved with mobile intensive care equipment to another part of the hospital for scans or other tests.

The doctors and nurses use electronic monitors to supervise many aspects of the patient's condition. There may be one large or several smaller monitors (looking like television sets) near the bedside. These are connected to the patient and the surrounding equipment with numerous wires and probes. The screens show a continual display of changing information on the state of the patient, including the temperature, the breathing rate, heart rate and blood pressure, the electrical activity of the heart, and the amount of oxygen in the lungs and in the blood.

Children admitted to an intensive care unit because of meningitis, or with septicaemia caused by meningococcal bacteria, are often so ill that they cannot breathe adequately on their own, and need help from a ventilator (often called the life support machine). This can partly or completely take over the work of breathing for a patient, who is attached to the machine by a tube passing down into the wind pipe, inserted through the mouth or nose. Children who need support from a ventilator generally have to be heavily sedated with tranquillisers and pain killers, and sometimes will be given medication to relax their muscles completely so that the ventilator can blow oxygen into the lungs most efficiently.

Nearly all the medications used in intensive care are given by intravenous drip into the bloodstream. On a regular hospital ward the drip is usually inserted into a vein in the hand or arm, but in the intensive care unit it is often necessary to deliver many drugs quickly, and the intravenous drips used on the regular ward are not designed for this use. A large-bore intravenous drip, called a central line, may be inserted into one of the large veins of the body, for example in the neck. Such a line is usually long enough to reach close to the heart, which ensures that the drugs are pumped round the body more effectively.

Babies and children who need intensive care are often too ill to feed normally. In some cases nutrition can be provided by dripping liquid feed into a fine tube, called a nasogastric tube, which has been passed down the nose directly into the stomach. In some circumstances when the stomach and intestines cannot absorb fluids, special feeds may be given through the central line directly into the bloodstream.

On a paediatric intensive care unit there are specialised doctors and nurses on duty all round the clock, ready to respond to emergencies whenever they occur. Each child will have one nurse by the bedside at all times, and the doctors are never far away. The team working in the unit will include paediatricians and other doctors, nurses, intensive care technicians, physiotherapists and a dietician. Each child is under the overall care of one consultant - the head of the unit or another specialist - and that doctor will always be available in emergencies, or by arrangement to discuss progress.

CHAPTER 5
What happens after meningitis?

Introduction

In the UK, nineteen out of twenty children with bacterial meningitis survive their infection. Many survivors of meningitis have got back virtually to normal by the time they are ready to go home from hospital, and go on to make a complete recovery *(plate 16, page 27)*. However, a few still have significant problems at the time of discharge from hospital, and though many of these get better over the next weeks or months, about one in ten will be left with some degree of permanent disability.

Temporary problems after meningitis.

The anxieties and the disruption of a family's routine that comes from having a child seriously ill in hospital often leave their mark for a while with difficult behaviour in the child. Tantrums are not uncommon, and the child may have nightmares, other sleep disturbance, or feeding problems. Children who are just gaining independence may temporarily regress a little - wanting to be carried everywhere, wetting the bed - but these things usually correct themselves within a week or two. It is quite common for adults who have had viral meningitis to complain of tiredness, irritability and reduced concentration for a while after the illness, but generally the problems are over within a month or two. Rarely, symptoms are more severe or long-drawn-out. Sufferers have sometimes found it difficult to get their problems taken seriously, as they seem outwardly well. They and their families have reported changes of character after viral meningitis, with aggressive behaviour, moodiness and learning difficulties. A very few have even feared that they are going mad. Fortunately even these distressing problems generally resolve with time.

In septicaemia caused by meningococcal bacteria, the skin in areas affected by the rash may be destroyed. Early on in the healing process a hard black scab covers the damaged area, but later this separates and new skin grows back. The area heals rather like a deep burn, to leave a scar *(plate 16, page 27)*. If large areas are damaged then skin grafts may be needed, but fortunately this is not common.

More serious problems after meningitis

One of the great fears in a case of meningitis is that the victim will be left with brain damage. In fact this only happens in about one in ten cases. Table 5 shows the rate with which different forms of this complication is seen.

Table 5. Outcome of bacterial meningitis

	Percentage of cases
Survivors of meningitis	95%
Survivors who recover entirely	85%
Survivors with some degree of brain damage	10%
including one or more of the following problems:	
Mild Hearing loss	5%
Severe Hearing loss	5%
Some degree of weakness or paralysis	4%
Fits	4%
Mild mental retardation (speech delay, slow learning)	2%
Severe mental retardation	2%

In the first days of treatment of a patient with meningitis or septicaemia caused by meningococcal bacteria, it may be almost impossible to predict whether, or how severely, a victim will be damaged. Even someone who is unconscious on life support for days may go on to make a full recovery (See Amy's story *(page 31)*. Long after discharge from hospital improvement is still to be expected, and there are many remarkable examples of recovery, as described for example in the continuation of Amanda's story.

In many cases the disabilities arising from the brain damage can be lessened by various kinds of therapy. Hearing aids or in severe cases, a cochlear implant (as described in the continuation of Edward's story later in this chapter), may relieve the commonest of the problems after meningitis - deafness. Physiotherapy, occupational therapy, speech therapy and special education may be needed in cases where brain damage is more severe, as described in the continuation of Amanda's story; and fits can usually be completely controlled with medication.

The damage that meningococcal bacteria cause in severe septicaemia can be very widespread. In a few cases there is such serious damage to skin and muscle that the victim will lose fingers or toes, or even part of a leg, as the result of gangrene. With plastic surgery, orthopaedic surgery and where needed, modern artificial limbs, these children can nevertheless be expected to lead very full, active lives.

Two examples of victims with persisting problems who needed longer term treatment are Amanda *(see page 45)* and Edward *(see page 39)*.

Amanda's Story (continued from page 46):

Amanda, aged 20, was saved by her uncle breaking the door down to get into her flat, where she was slipping into a coma from septicaemia caused by meningococcal bacteria.

Coming out of the coma, I remember being in a lot of discomfort and could not understand what had happened to me. It was a frightening experience as I could hardly see or speak and found it hard to move my arms and legs. Even in those early days I received physiotherapy, occupational therapy and speech therapy. I remember that the first words I spoke were to my mum and dad. "You can go now", I said. I think I was sick of the sight of them!!

I spent six weeks in the hospital and was then transferred to a rehabilitation unit for intensive therapy. That's when the reality of the situation hit me and I realised that what had happened to me wasn't going to go away.

My first day in the rehabilitation unit was not one I wish to remember. From being in my own separate room in the hospital to being put in a ward with others was very hard to adjust to. I remember sitting in that wheelchair and not being able to do a thing. From day one I was encouraged to do things for myself and believe you me it wasn't easy. I had to learn the basics all over again.

To enable me to make any progress I had to get intensive physiotherapy, occupational therapy and speech therapy. Just trying to feed and dress myself was very hard and very frustrating! My main aim was to get back on my feet and walk again. My speech was also very important to me and this, like everything else, took a long time.

After nine months in hospital I finally got home but things weren't easy. Adjusting to the outside world was very hard to do. Although I was being discharged my programme was not yet complete and I attended out-patients every week for eighteen months still making progress.

On being discharged from hospital I went back to live with my parents as I needed a lot of help and support. I went back to college on a part-time basis doing various different modules to help build up my confidence. I found it very hard to focus on other things, like college, because all I was interested in was getting back to normal.

I have been left partially sighted and my right side is considerably weaker than my left. Having been right handed before I am now learning to write again with my left hand. My walking still causes me problems and outside I use a stick.

Last year I made my biggest achievement towards getting my independence back again by moving into my own flat. I have just started another course of physiotherapy, so hopefully within time my walking will improve further. After three years I still find it a constant struggle and don't think I'll ever come to terms with what has happened to me. I get very down at times when I dwell on my situation and constantly think, "Why me?", but I am still optimistic about the future and remain determined to progress further....

Edward's Story (continued from page 39):

Edward, aged 15 months, had meningitis caused by pneumococcal bacteria. After three days in a coma on the high dependency unit, he regained consciousness.

When Edward was transferred back to the ward, after being in the high dependency unit for three days, we knew immediately something was still wrong. He was constantly crying, banging his head against the bars of the cot, not able to support his head, sit up or walk. When we were able to take him to the play area in an attempt to soothe him, we noticed he did not seem to be responding to his name or any of the noise making toys. The doctor told us that hearing can be affected in meningitis but it usually comes back, it was just a matter of time.

After one week in hospital we were advised to go home because of the way it was affecting Edward: he would be better off at home. He would be seen regularly in the outpatient department. Again we expressed our concern for his hearing, and we were told it would be tested about six weeks after the start of his illness.

Over the next few weeks things were not easy. Edward was banging his head on the floor or the nearest object. He had to learn to walk all over again. It took six weeks, and for months after that he had balance problems. His behaviour had changed completely and the head banging went on.

When Edward went for hearing tests the results were bad. He was found to be profoundly deaf in both ears. We were told about a new procedure for deaf children that might help Edward - cochlear implants - and he was referred to a specialist. Edward had a cochlear implant eighteen months later and it seems to have been a real success. He is now a very happy 4 year old who does not seem to have a care in the world. His behaviour has improved and there is no more frustration. He can make himself understood through sign and gesture. He goes to an integrated school with both deaf and hearing children for five mornings a week, and his speech is just beginning to come through.

It is still hard to believe he had meningitis as he had none of symptoms you are told to look out for. However, when his implant is switched off he is still deaf and that is reality.

Follow-up in the clinic after meningitis.

Most patients who have been discharged from hospital after meningitis are seen again in an outpatients' clinic. The main purpose of this visit is to check that recovery is complete or continuing, and to plan for the future management of any problems that might remain. A hearing test is usually arranged for about six weeks after the date of the infection. This will be carried out by a hearing specialist (an audiologist) with equipment that can detect even minor degrees of hearing loss in small children - something that may not be obvious even to parents. If hearing loss is found, arrangements will be made for long term follow-up, and the provision of any aids that may be needed. In those cases where there has been more extensive damage, the child may be referred to a specialist in child development. This is usually a paediatrician who works with a team of physiotherapists, educational psychologists, specialist health visitors and social workers to ensure that all appropriate help is provided.

The clinic visit also provides an opportunity to consider whether there might be any defect in the ability to fight infection which led to the child getting meningitis in the first place. Blood tests, and occasionally special X-rays, maybe needed to investigate this.

Loss of a child

Tragically, some children will die from meningitis or septicaemia in spite of receiving the best care available. Understandably there is much difficulty and often bitterness in coming to terms with this loss. In a desperate search for answers parents may come to blame themselves or others for failing to act quickly enough, or to make an early diagnosis. It is important for parents to have adequate time to air their views, and so arrangements are generally made for them to see the paediatric consultant who was in charge of the case for bereavement counselling. In cases where a post mortem examination was carried out, the results may be available and can also be discussed.

Support Organisations

There are many organisations which can help the victims of meningitis and their families (addresses and telephone numbers are given in the Appendix). Foremost among these in the UK are The Meningitis Research Foundation and The National Meningitis Trust. These organisations were each established by families who lost children to meningitis, and both have similar charitable aims and activities.

The Meningitis Research Foundation, whose members have helped in producing this book and to whom it is dedicated, was formed in 1989 by parents who lost their son to meningitis, and it has grown rapidly to a major national charity which in 1995 raised nearly £1,000,000 to fight this devastating disease. The Foundation operates in two main areas: information and awareness, and research. Provision of information and support are among the key activities of the Foundation. There is a round-the-clock telephone helpline which takes a very wide range of calls, from basic requests for information from the Public or the Press to calls from individuals with specific questions relating to their own experience. It has received calls from parents who are worried about a sick child, from the families of people who are critically ill in hospital, and not uncommonly from bereaved parents who simply need someone to listen. Support for families in crisis as a result of these devastating illnesses is provided, where desired, on a one-to-one basis. A member of the Foundation's trustees or staff may visit a family to offer support and information, to listen, and where appropriate to share experiences. The Foundation holds members' meetings around the country, so that families have an opportunity to come together and offer mutual support. The Foundation publishes a range of information resources on meningitis, and every autumn, when cases start to increase, there is a major information campaign. The Foundation, advised by an impartial panel of scientific and medical experts, also makes a substantial investment in the form of grants to scientists engaged in research into meningitis.

CHAPTER 6

Outbreaks: Preventing the Spread of Bacterial Meningitis

Infections caused by meningococcal bacteria

Whenever a case of meningococcal disease occurs, there is a worry that there may be further cases in those who were in close contact with the victim in the early stages of infection. Although some will probably be carrying the bacteria *(see page 56)*, the likelihood of their falling ill is very small indeed, but preventive treatment is offered to all those who are at risk. These are: the family living in the same house as the victim, anyone else who slept overnight in the house during the ten days previously, and girlfriends and boyfriends ("kissing contacts" - kisses on the mouth, not just a kiss on the cheek). All these people will be offered a short course of antibiotic medicine to kill meningococcal bacteria that may be lurking in their noses and throats. This has the important effect of minimising the spread of the bacteria amongst individuals who may be at risk. However, although the antibiotic will destroy the bacteria in the nose and throat, it is not sufficient to kill bacteria if they have entered the bloodstream. Therefore the contacts who are given antibiotic should also be warned that they should go to the doctor promptly if they feel unwell. If the case was caused by a strain of meningococcal bacteria against which there is a vaccine (see chapter 8), then this same group will also be offered vaccination for longer term protection. The protective effect of vaccination develops at 7-10 days after the injection. More distant contacts, such as friends, neighbours or people who visited the house for short periods in the days before the victim fell ill, should be warned that the case has occurred, but the risk to them is so low that they do not generally need antibiotic medicine or vaccine.

When a case occurs in a child who attends play group or school, the most important thing is that all the parents are given adequate information. Usually this will be in a joint letter from the head teacher and local public health doctor. In this it will be stated that a case has occurred, that the chance of spread to other children is extremely small, but that the GP should be contacted for advice on any feverish illness against the very slight possibility that it might be a second case. The Health Education Authority/Department of Health and the meningitis support charities (the Meningitis Research Foundation and the National Meningitis Trust) all produce excellent leaflets describing the signs and symptoms of meningitis and septicaemia, with colour photographs of the spots, and such a leaflet may be included in the letter. In general, classmates are not given antibiotic medicine, although any children who have been particularly close to the victim may be.

If a second case of meningococcal disease occurs within four weeks in the same play-group, nursery or primary school, all the children and the staff are given antibiotic medicine, and vaccinated if appropriate. In a secondary school or college setting, every attempt is made to work out the way in which infection may have passed from one person to another, and all those who might be involved are offered antibiotics. Again, if vaccine could be effective it would be given too for longer term protection. If both victims are in the same hall of residence at college, or in the same class or study group, or share some other activity in common, then all the others in the same group may be offered the medicine. However, it is often very difficult to know where to draw the line when, for example, two children in different year groups who have no lessons in common are affected. A short course of antibiotics is of very little value in preventing infection if the germs are circulating widely in the community, ready to cause infection as soon as the antibiotics have been finished. The most important thing again is that information is distributed widely, so that anyone who should become ill is seen without delay by their doctor. If the strain of meningococcal bacteria responsible for the outbreak turns out to be one against which there is a vaccine, the public health doctor will arrange vaccinations to protect everyone in the school or college.

Hib meningitis

Before the introduction of Hib vaccine in 1992 (see chapter 8), there were the same worries about the spread of Hib meningitis as there are now about meningococcal infection. Small children in contact with a case were at risk, and protective antibiotics were prescribed in much the same way. The problem has virtually disappeared with Hib vaccination. If a case ever does occur and there is any other unvaccinated child under 4 years old in the household, everyone in the household is offered antibiotics to kill any germs they might be carrying, and unimmunised children are offered vaccination as soon as possible.

Other forms of meningitis

No other forms of meningitis caused by bacteria are known to cause outbreaks in the community. Although pneumococcal bacteria, responsible for pneumococcal meningitis, are carried in the nose and throat like meningococcal or Hib bacteria, contacts of a case of meningitis virtually never develop the disease. No antibiotic treatment or vaccination is necessary for contacts.

CHAPTER 7
Travel and meningitis

Travellers in Europe, North America and Australasia

The risk of developing meningitis on holiday anywhere in Europe, North America or Australasia is extremely low, the same as it would be at home in the UK. As meningitis is a seasonal disease, and in Europe and North America generally even rarer in the summer than it is in the winter, the chances of coming down with the infection while on summer holiday are very small indeed. However it can happen, and coinciding as the summer holidays do with a time when the media are hungry for news, cases make a big splash. Several cases of meningitis and septicaemia caused by meningococcal bacteria occurred in visitors to the Mediterranean island of Majorca in the early summer of 1996. British newspapers carried the story for days, and there was a lot of anxiety about the risks to other holiday makers - the dangers of mingling in the hotels, visiting discos, using swimming pools and so on. In fact the risk was no different from that at home, and the same precautions routinely taken in England to prevent the spread of infection (see Chapter 6) were effectively used in Majorca to stop further cases occurring.

Travellers in Africa, Asia and South America

As long-haul holidays to exotic places have become increasingly popular and affordable, meningitis caused by meningococcal bacteria has to be added to the list of diseases against which travellers may need to be vaccinated. The particular risk is of infection caused by serogroup A meningococcal bacteria, and back-packers, hitch-hikers, and those living in local conditions rather than in tourist hotels are most likely to be exposed, during large outbreaks which occur regularly in the countries of the meningitis belt of Africa (Figure 5). This is a broad irregular band across the continent south of the Sahara desert, extending from Senegal in the west to Kenya in the east, where outbreaks of meningitis and septicaemia caused by serogroup A meningococcal bacteria occur each dry season (which starts some time between December and February and continues until the onset of the rains in May or June). While serogroup A strains of meningococcal bacteria only causes a handful of cases if any in the UK each year, there are thousands of cases and hundreds of deaths virtually every year in the meningitis belt. About every ten years there are particularly large epidemics. The most recent was in 1996, when the epidemic was described as the worst in living memory. The World Health Organisation issued a bulletin in July 1996, noting at least 140,000 cases of meningitis and 15,000 deaths in Africa in the first six months of the year.

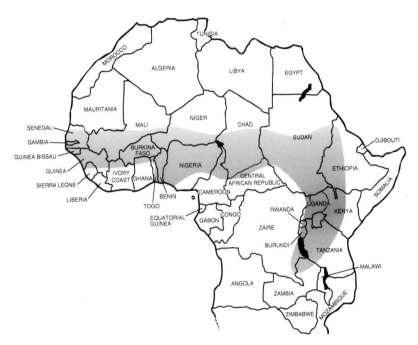

Figure 5. The meningitis belt of Africa.

The meningitis belt of Africa. The shaded area shows countries in which there may be seasonal outbreaks of meningitis caused by meningococcal bacteria. The boundaries of the meningitis belt are not precisely defined, and the risk is seasonal and will vary depending on the precise destination. Travellers should seek up-to-date advice about the need for vaccination in good time before setting off.

Countries outside Africa for which meningococcal vaccine is sometimes recommended to travellers include: *in Asia*: Bangladesh, Bhutan, India (especially in the area around New Delhi), Myanmar (Burma), Nepal, Pakistan,the Philippines, and Saudi Arabia (required for pilgrims during the Hajj); and *in South America*: Brazil. As for travellers to sub-Saharan Africa, up-to-date advice about the need for vaccination should be obtained in good time before setting off.

During the Hajj (pilgrimage to Mecca, Saudi Arabia), travellers can be very crowded together, and outbreaks of infection caused by serogroup A meningococcal bacteria have occurred. In 1987, 23 cases of meningitis were reported in pilgrims from the UK or their close contacts. Since 1988 the Saudi Arabian Authorities have required pilgrims to be immunised against infection caused by meningococcal bacteria. They must produce a certificate to this effect, dated not less than ten days, but not more than three years, before their arrival in Saudi Arabia.

Vaccination for travellers: meningococcal vaccination

Two vaccines are currently (1997) licensed in the UK for protecting travellers against infection caused by meningococcal bacteria. These each contain purified material from the outer coat of the bacteria, and provide cover against serogroup A and serogroup C strains. There is no protection against serogroup B strains, which are responsible for most cases that arise in the UK *(see page 64)*.

General practitioners can prescribe and inject meningococcal vaccine. A charge may be made for this. Only a single dose is required, and protection starts from 5 to 7 days after the injection. However, you should consult your doctor in good time before you travel, as other vaccinations may also be advisable and these may need to be spaced out over a few weeks. In particular, travellers anywhere should be sure that their tetanus and polio immunisation is up-to-date.

More than 9 out of 10 vaccinated adults are protected against both serogroup A and serogroup C meningococcal infection by the single dose, and this protection lasts for three to five years. The vaccines are less effective in children. In children over 2 years old, immunity is usually gone by about two years after injection. The under 2s do not (in most cases) respond to the serogroup C part of the vaccine, though all but the youngest (under 3 months old) should make a response to the serogroup A part, which is the most important for travellers. Babies aged between three months and 2 years travelling to a high risk area should therefore be given the vaccine, and the dose repeated at around 2 years of age if continued protection is needed.

Serious reactions are very rare indeed. About one in ten people may have a mild reaction of discomfort, redness or mild swelling at the injection site starting shortly after vaccination and lasting for a day or two. Children, more commonly than adults, may have a short period of fever.

There are some special situations in which meningitis vaccination should not be taken. Vaccination should be delayed if you are unwell with an acute feverish illness. Anyone who has had a severe reaction to meningococcal vaccine in the past should not be given a further dose. There is no reason to believe that meningococcal vaccine is unsafe during pregnancy, but it is generally felt prudent to avoid vaccinations during pregnancy unless there is a clear need. Necessary travel to a high-risk area would be justification for vaccination. Meningococcal vaccine can usually be given safely to HIV-positive individuals.

Vaccination for travellers: Hib vaccination

If young babies are being taken abroad, it is very important that the complete set of three Hib immunisations is given as it would be at home (in the UK, at 2, 3 and 4 months of age), to protect against meningitis caused by Hib bacteria. As there are different formulations made by different manufacturers, it may be that the course of injections was started at home with a brand not available abroad. This does not appear to matter, and the course should be completed with whatever vaccine is licensed in the country you are staying.

Meningitis vaccination for travellers.

For up-to-date information:

- Your GP, a travel clinic, or your travel agent may be able to advise on the need for meningococcal vaccination.

- Booklet "HEALTH advice for travellers". Obtainable free from Health Literature Line (freephone call 0800 555777)

- Hospital for Tropical Diseases: Travel Clinic Health line: Phone 0839 337733

Leave plenty of time before travelling to arrange for any vaccinations that may be needed.

Chapter 8
Meningitis Vaccines: the present and the future

Two of the vaccines that are currently offered routinely to all children in the UK prevent varieties of meningitis.

Hib vaccine

The first vaccine to protect children against bacterial meningitis was Hib vaccine, first used in the mid 1980s in the USA. The first version of the vaccine to be developed could only protect children over the age of 2 years,

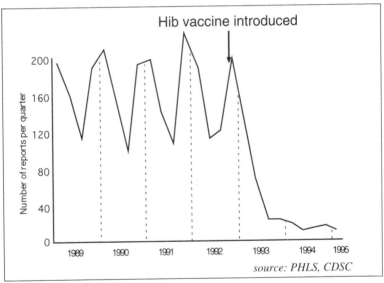

source: PHLS, CDSC

Figure 6. Quarterly reports of cases of Hib meningitis and septicaemia, 1988 - 1995.
The saw-tooth pattern reflects the seasonal variation, with many cases in the winter and fewer in the summer. On the introduction of the Hib vaccine at the end of 1992, there was a sudden and sustained fall in the number of cases to a very low level.

but a newer version was soon available which was also effective in babies. This was introduced in the UK in autumn of 1992 and has made a tremendous impact (Figure 6).

Until the vaccine was introduced, Hib caused about four in every ten cases of bacterial meningitis in England and Wales, about 1500 cases each year. Well over half the children were under two years old, and in about one case in twenty the child died. Since 1982, all children have been offered Hib vaccine at the same time as the routine diphtheria, tetanus, whooping cough and polio vaccinations at 2, 3 and 4 months of age. There has been such a dramatic reduction in the number of cases, down to only 46 in England and Wales in the year to mid-1996, that there is a realistic hope that Hib meningitis will disappear altogether.

Measles, mumps and rubella vaccine (MMR)

Infection with an important cause of viral meningitis, the mumps virus, can nearly always be prevented with the measles, mumps and rubella (german measles) vaccine (MMR), offered to all children in the UK at 12-15 months of age and again at school entry. The vaccine contains greatly weakened strains of the three viruses, and induces immunity by causing very mild infection. This is usually not apparent at all, but it may be marked by a day or so of mild fever, irritability and a slight rash a fortnight or so after the injection. It is not doing the MMR vaccine justice, however, to present it simply as the means of preventing cases of mumps meningitis. Mumps has other complications including sterility, measles has many miserable complications, including life-threatening inflammation of the brain in about one in a thousand cases, while rubella can cause devastating brain damage to babies in the womb. All these terrible problems can be avoided with MMR vaccine.

Vaccines to protect against meningitis and septicaemia caused by meningococcal and pneumococcal bacteria.

Meningococcal vaccines

Now that Hib meningitis cases are so rare, meningococcal bacteria are the leading cause of meningitis and septicaemia in the UK. Two main varieties cause nearly all the disease: serogroup B (causing seven out of ten cases) and serogroup C (three out of ten cases). In some parts of the world, although not in the UK, serogroup A strains of meningococcal bacteria cause vast numbers of cases (see chapter 7).

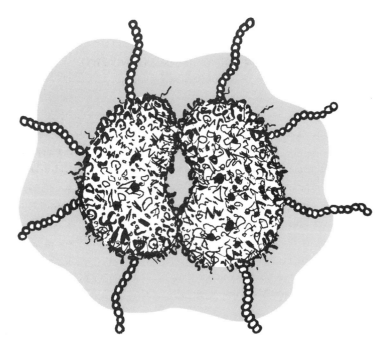

Figure 7. Meningococcal bacteria
Two meningococcal bacteria are shown, enveloped in a thick layer of slimy outer coat material (shading). Under the coat, the surface of the bacteria is studded with many different components, some of them elongated fibres that protrude through the coating.

The struggle to make really effective vaccines to prevent meningococcal infections is still a major challenge for researchers, but there is a lot of optimism that this will be solved very soon, at least for some varieties of the bacteria. There are already vaccines that provide some protection against infections with the serogroup A and C varieties, but these only work well in children over the age of two, just like the early sort of Hib vaccine did. Newer versions, which should be as good as the present Hib vaccine, have been undergoing trials through 1996. Preliminary data suggest that these should be highly effective, and once introduced into the UK vaccine programme, will prevent 500 or more cases of meningitis and septicaemia, with 50 or more deaths, caused by serogroup C meningococcal bacteria each year.

Vaccines that protect against infections caused by serogroup C and serogroup A meningococcal bacteria are manufactured from the slimy outer coat that surrounds each organism (figure 7). Such vaccines are themselves harmless, but if they are injected into a person they stimulate the body's immune system to protect against infection caused by the bacteria from which they are made. Unfortunately, it is not possible to make a vaccine from the outer coat of the common serogroup B strains. Different components studding the bacterial surface underneath the coat, or poking out through it (figure 7), have been studied to see if they can be used instead to make a vaccine, but the problem has been to find one or a set of these components which between them are present in all strains of serogroup B bacteria. Unlike the slimy outer coat, which is a constant feature of all strains, the other components are very variable. No experimental vaccines based on these components have yet been developed that can protect against all the different strains of serogroup B meningococcal bacteria that are causing cases of disease.

A possible solution has been suggested by researchers in Cuba, where an urgent hunt for a vaccine was inspired by an epidemic of meningococcal infection in the 1970s. Instead of trying to identify a single component of the bacteria to make into a vaccine, it was reasoned that a vaccine made of many different components might protect against many different strains at once. As meningococcal bacteria divide, little bubbles of the outer surface, known as blebs, break off from the surface. This can be seen happening in photographs of bacteria taken at high magnification with an electron microscope *(Figure 8)*.

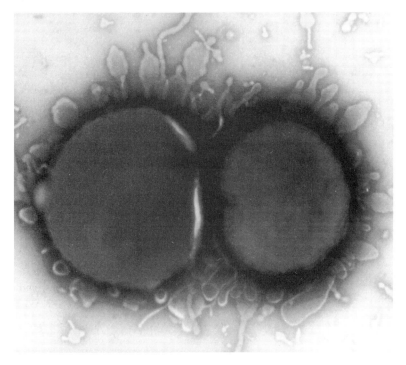

Figure 8. Meningococcal bacteria.
A hugely magnified photograph of bacteria dividing, showing the production of blebs appearing like bubbles off the surface.

As each bleb is itself covered with a wide range of different surface components from the bacteria, injection of a vaccine made from blebs could lead to protection against infections caused by many different strains of serogroup B meningococcal bacteria. Purified blebs that may be used in a vaccine have been made by researchers in Cuba, Norway and Holland. Some trials of such vaccines in children of different ages have produced promising results, and if they can be shown to protect the youngest children at greatest risk, (the under 1s), there is every prospect that larger trials will shortly follow.

Pneumococcal vaccines

A vaccine made from a mixture of outer coat material extracted from twenty three different strains of pneumococcal bacteria can give useful protection against infection, but once again in its present form it only works in children over two years old and in adults. In the UK a vaccine of this sort is offered to some people who are at particular risk of infection, such as those whose spleens do not work properly (see chapter 3). There is a major practical problem in modifying the vaccine to work in babies by using the same approach as that so successfully employed in the case of Hib. In contrast to the single variety of Hib, there are nearly 100 different varieties of pneumococcal bacteria, and a different vaccine would be needed to protect against each one. While only six or seven strains predominate as causes of disease in any one country, different countries have different sets, and also this pattern can change over time. Therefore a vaccine preventing infections caused by one set of strains might only be useful in some countries, and would have only a limited useful life span. Not withstanding this complication, vaccine companies are developing products along these lines, containing a mixture of modified outer coat material from anything between six and eleven different varieties of pneumococcal bacteria, but it is possible that they will be so expensive that only the wealthy countries will be able to afford to introduce them. Although such a vaccine will prevent some cases of meningitis, its main value is likely to be in the prevention of the commoner infections caused by pneumococcal bacteria - pneumonia, and less serious conditions like ear infections.

Conclusion

Meningitis is a rare disease. Because cases can be dramatic, meningitis has a high profile in the media - quite out of proportion to the two thousand or so of the serious cases that actually occur each year. Most people's lives will never be touched by meningitis in themselves, their friends or their loved ones.

Vaccines will one day be available to protect against nearly all the common causes of bacterial meningitis. We already have the Hib vaccine which has been very successful in almost eradicating meningitis caused by Hib bacteria. Vaccines against meningococcal and pneumococcal bacteria are on the horizon. However, for the immediate future there is no way that infections caused by these bacteria can be prevented by vaccination. Therefore, the important thing is to be able to recognise the early signs and symptoms of these diseases. This can be life saving. Cases that are recognised and treated in time are nearly always completely cured.

Appendix - Support Organisations

Association for all speech impaired
children (AFASIC)

347, Central Markets,
Smithfield, London EC1A 9NH
(0171 236 3632)

Association for Children with Hand
or Arm deficiency (REACH)

12, Wilson Way, Earlsbarton,
Northants. NN6 0NZ
(0160 4811041)

British Deaf Association

1, Worship Street,
London EC2A 2AB
(0171 588 3520)

British Epilepsy Association

Anstey House,
40 Hanover Square,
Leeds LS3 1BE (01532 439393)

Meningitis Research Foundation

13, High Street, Thornbury,
Bristol BS12 2AE
(01454 281811).
HELPLINE: 01454 413344

National Deaf Children's Society

15, Dufferin Street,
London EC1Y 8PD
(0171 250 0123)

National Meningitis Trust

Fern House, Bath Road, Stroud,
Gloucestershire GL5 3TJ
(01453 751738)
HELPLINE: 0345 538118

National Portage Association	50, Orchard Hill, Little Billing, Northampton NN3 4AG (01604 407977)
Royal National Institute for the Blind	224, Great Portland Street, London W1N 6AA (0171 388 1266)
Royal National Institute for the Deaf	19-23 Featherstone Street, London EC1Y 8SL (0171 296 8000)
Royal Society for mentally-handicapped children and adults (MENCAP)	MENCAP National Centre, 123 Golden Lane, London EC1Y ORT (0171 454 0454)

Glossary

aciclovir	a medicine which will inactivate some sorts of viruses including herpes.
antibiotic	a medicine which kills bacteria.
antibodies	Proteins in the blood which are produced by the immune system (*qv*) to protect against infection.
antiviral drug	a medicine, such as aciclovir, which is effective against viruses.
bacteria	germs which cause different sorts of infections including meningitis.
barrier nursing	precautions taken while caring for a patient to ensure that infection cannot be passed on to others.
bleb	bubble-like structures that bud off the outer surface of meningococcal bacteria as they divide *(see Fig 8, page 102)*.
blood poisoning	*see* septicaemia.
cerebrospinal fluid	the fluid surrounding the brain and spinal cord which acts as a cushion to protect them *(see Fig 1, page 54-55)*.
cerebrospinal meningitis	*see* meningitis.
chicken pox	a very common childhood infection, caused by a virus known as varicella virus.
coliform	bacteria which usually inhabit the digestive tract harmlessly, but can sometimes cause infections, including meningitis in newborn babies.
coma	the state of being unconscious.

complement	a family of proteins in the blood which together with antibody *(qv)* form an important part of the body's defence against bacterial infection. Complement proteins are particularly important in fighting meningococcal infection.
convulsion	*see* fit.
CAT scan	*see* CT scan.
central line	a large intravenous drip *(qv)* which is inserted into one of the large veins of the body - often at the base of the neck or in the chest wall - so that medication and fluids can be given.
cochlear implant	a special type of hearing aid which is inserted deep inside the ear by a surgeon and may help people who have been left deaf by meningitis.
Computed Tomography scan	*see* CT scan.
CT scan	a specialised X-ray investigation in which a series of X-ray pictures, taken in rapid succession, are processed by computer to create an image of the interior of the body *(see plate 13, page 26, and Figure 4, page 78).*
enterovirus	a family of viruses which cause several different types of infection - most commonly diarrhoea or a cold/sore throat, but occasionally meningitis. polio virus is a dangerous variety of enterovirus: polio infection is preventable by immunisation.
fit	the result of scrambled brain-wave activity, which results in loss of consciousness, and stiffening or jerking of the arms and legs. Among possible triggers for a fit are: fever (particularly in small children between the ages of six months and five years); and meningitis. See box, page 15.
fontanelle	the soft spot on the top of a baby's head where the bones of the skull have not yet completely grown together.

germs	bacteria and viruses.
German Measles	a common virus infection, also known as rubella. German measles is preventable with the MMR vaccine *(qv)*.
glass test	a useful test that can be done at home to check if spots or a rash have features typical of meningococcal infection: see page 18.
GP	general practitioner or family doctor.
Group B streptococcal	bacteria which commonly inhabit the digestive tract and genital region of adults, doing no harm. On rare occasions they can cause infections in newborn babies, including meningitis.
Hib	A type of bacteria which is an important cause of infection, including meningitis, in humans. These infections are now preventable with Hib vaccine *(see page 98)*.
herpes	a virus which can cause cold sores (common), genital herpes (common) and meningitis (rare). Infections can be treated with aciclovir *(qv)*.
high dependency unit	a special hospital ward, or part of a ward, where a patient's condition can be monitored closely. Generally if life support is needed a patient would be transferred to an intensive care unit (see chapter 4).
immune system	The organs and blood cells which work together to detect and fight infection.
immunisation	use of vaccines *(qv)* to prevent infections.
inflammation	redness, swelling, heat and discomfort or pain resulting from damage to cells anywhere in the body.
intensive care unit	special hospital ward where a patient's condition can be monitored very closely, and where life support can be provided (see chapter 4).

intravenous drip — A fine plastic tube inserted into a vein using a needle, through which fluids and medication can be given straight into the bloodstream.

kissing contact — a person kissed on the lips by someone later developing meningitis *(see page 90)*.

Listeria — a type of bacteria that can contaminate some foods such as paté and which has been the cause of some cases of meningitis in newborn babies.

lumbar puncture — a test for meningitis which involves taking a small amount of cerebrospinal fluid *(qv)* from the base of the spine to be examined for signs of infection *(see Fig 1, page 54-55; Fig 3, page 76; plate 9, page 24)*.

measles — a virus infection, prevented by the MMR vaccine.

meninges — the coverings of the brain and spinal cord.

meningitis — inflammation of the coverings of the brain; bacteria and viruses cause bacterial meningitis and viral meningitis respectively.

meningococcal — the type of bacteria most commonly found causing bacterial meningitis in the UK; also the cause of meningococcal septicaemia.

middle ear — the space behind the ear drum. The is the part that is usually involved in an ear infection.

MMR — measles, mumps and rubella vaccine *(see page 99)*.

MRI scan — An MRI (magnetic resonance imaging) scan is similar to a CT scan *(qv)* in the picture it can give of the brain or other internal organs of the body, but the pictures are produced through use of a powerful magnetic field instead of X-rays. Sometimes referred to as NMR scan.

mumps virus — the virus responsible for the infection of the same name, which can also cause meningitis. Infection is prevented by MMR vaccine *(qv)*.

paediatrician	doctor who specialises in childhood illnesses.
paracetamol	a widely-used medicine which brings down the temperature and also relieves pain.
penicillin	one of the first antibiotics to be discovered, still very effective for treatment of some bacterial infections including some sorts of meningitis.
photophobia	literally, "fear of light"; a sign of meningitis (see chapter 1).
pneumococcal	the second commonest kind of bacteria causing meningitis in the UK after meningococcal bacteria.
polio	*see* enterovirus
seizure	*see* fit
septicaemia	also known as blood poisoning. In this condition bacteria multiply in the blood and spread all over the body to cause widespread damage.
septic arthritis	bacterial infection in a joint.
septic screen	a series of tests to look for infection (usually including blood tests, urine tests and a lumbar puncture *(qv))*.
serogroup	grouping of different strains of meningococcal bacteria according to the type of slimy outer coat which they possess.
spinal cord	an complex bundle of nerve cells and fibres extending down from the brain, protected by the bones of the spine, from which nerves pass out all over the body *(see Fig 1, page 54-55).*
spleen	an organ tucked in under the ribs on the left side of the body. The part of the immune system particularly involved in removing and destroying bacteria which have got into the bloodstream.

the big three meningitis bacteria — the three commonest causes of bacterial meningitis in the UK: meningococcal, pneumococcal and Hib bacteria.

unpasteurised — untreated by pasteurisation (a method used in the food industry to ensure that germs in foodstuffs are killed).

vaccine — A preparation of weakened or inactivated germs, or components of germs, which can be used to prevent future infections: e.g. MMR vaccine (*qv*) (containing weakened germs) and Hib vaccine (containing a component of the Hib bacteria) (see chapter 8).

vaccination — prevention of infections by giving a vaccine.

virus — minute germ, smaller than bacteria, responsible for many different kinds of infection, including meningitis.